"*Yoga for Emotional T* **MAY** - gap in the trauma and recovery literature. Anyone who is working to heal from past trauma will benefit from reading this book. Then, following the easy instructions for yoga poses will move their recovery in a new way. Well written and easily understood."

—**Charles Whitfield, MD**, author of *Not Crazy: You May Not be Mentally Ill* and *Wisdom to Know the Difference*, and **Barbara Harris Whitfield, RT, CMT**, author of *The Natural Soul, Victim to Survivor*, and *Thriver*

"To be alive in the twentyfirst century is to be traumatized, but we need not stay traumatized. Our age is witnessing an efflorescence of methods to eliminate suffering and move to a place of joy, fulfillment, and serenity. The NurrieStearns are leading the way."

—**Larry Dossey, MD**, author of *Healing Words* and *One Mind*

"You don't have to have a history of trauma to benefit from this manual of practices from the yoga tradition, but if you do, *Yoga for Emotional Trauma* is essential reading. The NurrieStearns write with compassion and understanding about the journey home to your true nature, the place that has never been sullied by your trauma. The NurrieStearns write clearly, humbly describing their own recovery from trauma along with the recovery stories of the many clients with whom they have worked. Thank you NurrieStearns for giving us in clear and readable prose, the brain science that explains the effects of trauma and how yoga can help us recover."

—**Amy Weintraub**, founder of the LifeForce Yoga Healing Institute, and author of *Yoga for Depression* and *Yoga Skills for Therapists*

"This is simply a fantastic book. It captures the full spectrum of practical knowledge of yoga and makes it accessible for all of us so we can use this ancient knowledge and proven practice for healing our body, mind, and spirit. Without overwhelming the reader, the book encourages us to try out a number of thoughtful compassionate and gentle exercises to soothe and harmonize all three aspects of ourselves: body, mind, and spirit."

—**Georg Eifert, PhD**, Chapman University Professor Emeritus of Psychology and coauthor of the *Mindfulness and Acceptance Workbook for Anxiety*

"Margaret Mitchell once wrote: 'Every problem has two handles. You can grab it by the handle of fear, or the handle of hope.' This book has a firm grasp on the handle of hope. This book offers a gentle, timetested, nurturing approach to guide the reader through their recovery from trauma. It is a muchneeded balm for a wounded world."

—**Henry Emmons, MD**, integrative psychiatrist and author of *The Chemistry of Joy*, *The Chemistry of Calm* and *The Chemistry of Joy Workbook*

"Yoga teachers, students, and even folks new to the idea of yoga will benefit from the stories and information in this thoughtful book. The healing power of yoga is vast and endless both physically and emotionally. The authors have done a wonderful job of explaining how it works with easytounderstand true stories and references to science. I appreciate this work and plan to share it with all of my students and teacher trainees. We can help so many people, and we can begin with ourselves."

—**Desiree Rumbaugh**, certified yoga instructor

yoga for emotional trauma

meditations and
practices for healing pain
and suffering

Mary NurrieStearns
Rick NurrieStearns

New Harbinger Publications, Inc.

Publisher's Note

This publication is designed to provide accurate and authoritative information in regard to the subject matter covered. It is sold with the understanding that the publisher is not engaged in rendering psychological, financial, legal, or other professional services. If expert assistance or counseling is needed, the services of a competent professional should be sought.

Distributed in Canada by Raincoast Books

Copyright © 2013 by Mary NurrieStearns & Rick NurrieStearns
         New Harbinger Publications, Inc.
         5674 Shattuck Avenue
         Oakland, CA 94609
         www.newharbinger.com

Yoga posture photographs copyright © Carol Curry, Studio-Curry.com, 2012.

Illustration of seven chakras Copyright © Surabhi25/Shutterstock.com, 2012. Used under license from Shutterstock.com.

Acquired by Jess O'Brien; Cover design by Amy Shoup;
Text design by Michele Waters-Kermes; Edited by Marisa Solís

Library of Congress Cataloging-in-Publication Data

NurrieStearns, Mary.
  Yoga for emotional trauma : meditations and practices for healing pain and suffering / Mary NurrieStearns, LCSW, RYT, Rick NurrieStearns.
     pages cm
  Summary: "In Yoga for Emotional Trauma, a psychotherapist and a meditation teacher present a yogic approach to emotional trauma by instructing readers to apply mindful awareness, breathing, yoga postures, and mantras to their emotional and physical pain"-- Provided by publisher.
  Includes bibliographical references.
  ISBN 978-1-60882-642-1 (pbk.) -- ISBN 978-1-60882-643-8 (pdf e-book) -- ISBN 978-1-60882-644-5 (epub) 1. Psychic trauma--Alternative treatment. 2. Post-traumatic stress disorder--Alternative treatment. 3. Hatha yoga. 4. Self-care, Health. I. NurrieStearns, Rick. II. Title.
  RC552.T7N87 2013
  616.85'21062--dc23

                    2013014283

Printed in the United States of America

15 14 13   10 9 8 7 6 5 4 3 2 1   First printing

contents

acknowledgments

althought we wrote the words, this book reflects the lives and efforts of many great minds and hearts. To begin, we bow in gratitude to those individuals, living and dead, whose compassion has opened our hearts and who have taught us about meditation and yoga. Included in this group are luminaries such as Paramhansa Yogananda, Sri Nisargadatta Maharaj, Ramana Maharshi, Mahatma Gandhi, Father Thomas Keating, and Thich Nhat Hanh, along with less famous yoga and meditation teachers who have instructed us over the years, as well as strangers with big hearts who, without knowing their impact, have touched our lives and strengthened our faith in the resiliency of the human spirit.

We continue by thanking our community of family, friends, yoga students, and retreatants. Your dedication to healing has taught us more than you realize. Your stories of courage, love, and perseverance fill our hearts and the pages of this book. A special thanks to Meghan Donnelly for believing in our work and opening your yoga studio to us.

We thank New Harbinger Publications, especially editors Jess O'Brien and Nicola Skidmore, for making this book possible and for skillfully guiding us through the writing process. Your wise counsel kept the book on track and made it readable. We also express gratitude to Marisa Solís. Thank you for making the copyediting process as easy as possible for us as you finely tuned the book.

We thank those who have studied the effects of trauma on body and mind. Your efforts have helped us understand what trauma does to us and what is needed to heal from trauma. We also thank those who have researched the effects of yoga practices on the body and mind. Your work has helped to explain how and why yoga frees its practitioners from the grips of trauma. We reference you throughout the book. We do want to pay tribute to Peter Levine and Bessel van der Kolk for making extraordinary advancements in the treatment of emotional trauma. We also acknowledge Kenneth Pargament, whose research has verified the power of spirituality in psychological healing.

Special thanks go to the following people: to yogini Kristie Hale for beautifully modeling the yoga poses; to artist Carol Curry for taking great photographs; to Barbara Whitfield and Ellie Finlay for reading the manuscript, giving emotional sustenance, and offering helpful feedback; to Hal Zina Bennett for providing constructive criticism early in the writing process.

Finally, we thank our family and friends, including our four-legged ones. Your comforting presence, encouraging words, patience with our inattentiveness to you, wonderful gifts of food, discussions about the book, and overall loving support sustained us during this year of writing.

introduction

Each one has to find his peace from within. And peace to be real must be unaffected by outside circumstances.

—Mahatma Gandhi

When Rick NurrieStearns was in his twenties he called himself a spiritual seeker and traveled the world, studying Eastern philosophy and ways of living that would help him find authenticity and happiness. When Mary NurrieStearns was in her twenties she immersed herself in professional studies, thinking that advanced degrees were her ticket to a better life. Wanting something different in life than what we had been exposed to, we wanted to feel normal, possibly even happy. Even though our motives were unclear to us at the time, and our paths were different, we figured that having the right knowledge and doing the correct things would make us into good enough people. We had an underlying belief that everything, ourselves included, would be okay once we figured out what standards we had to achieve.

Young and idealistic, we were willing to work hard for fulfillment. Happiness was something to strive for, to be experienced in the future when we had made ourselves worthy. Rick's travels gave him invaluable exposure and Mary's studies gave her great opportunities. While travel and graduate school contributed significantly to each of our lives, they were not the direct routes to healing and happiness that we thought they would be.

Neither of us knew that contentment does not come as the result of treating yourself as an imperfect being who needs serious self-improvement. We did not know that deep inside we were already whole and worthy. We certainly did not know that peace comes from within. Then the wonderful healing practices and philosophy of yoga came into our lives. Yoga taught us that we are born with self-worth and do not have to manufacture it, that we have experiences but are not defined by them, that we have thoughts but we are not the contents of our thoughts. Yoga showed us how to go beneath the realms of thoughts and experiences into rich interior stillness, from which contentment arises. Yoga has not made our personalities perfect, nor prevented us from experiencing occasional distress or from making mistakes, but it has helped us find peace and given us skills to deal with the ups and downs of life.

Yoga is a tradition of tremendous breadth and depth, and we are neither yoga experts nor scholars. We are practitioners who credit yoga practices with profound personal healing. Accordingly, this is a self-help book, not an academic one. This book has a personal tone. We share examples, many from our own lives, so that you can read, firsthand, how powerfully healing yoga is. We also want you to feel supported by us. We do not know about your trauma, but we do know how trauma has touched our lives.

This book addresses what trauma does to the body and mind, and how and why yoga practices are so healing for those of us who have suffered from trauma. We include science, yoga philosophy, physiology, and research for a couple of reasons. Some of you are yoga teachers and health care professionals who want a body of knowledge about yoga as a healing modality. Also, a certain amount of information is healing, as it helps you to understand your personal experience. The educational components enhance the book's primary purpose as a self-help book to help you find inner peace.

We wholeheartedly encourage you to give yoga a chance. This book is filled with yoga practices that release trauma from your body, show you how to take care of your emotions, teach you to relate to rather than be consumed by thoughts, and focus your attention on your priorities and present-day life. Throughout the book, we present the fundamental teaching of yoga—which is that you and your life is a blessing.

chapter 1

healing involves compassion

It takes tender care and respect to heal the wounds of trauma. Compassion, which arises out of the recognition that human life is sacred, gives deep care and respect. In fact, compassion is a core component of healing, in part because each practice of compassion is an act of treating yourself with basic human decency.

In this chapter we address the role of compassion in healing trauma. We also teach you many compassionate practices that melt grief, restore self-worth, and help increase the joy in your life.

Opening Your Heart

Betrayal is central to many of the traumas that occur between people. Trust is breached, an agreement is broken, a responsibility is forsaken, or perhaps someone is treated as subhuman. In fact, maltreatment is degrading and often oppressive. It is not surprising then that, according to Marylene Cloitre (2006), issues with safety, trust, connections, self-esteem, and control are primary outcomes of childhood trauma. How could it be otherwise? Children's needs for safety, affection, recognition, and mastery are necessary for healthy development. The outcomes of adult traumas are not so different. Not only do adult traumas bring up unresolved childhood issues, but betrayal is painful and disruptive, uprooting, at least temporarily, the sense that you and life are okay. Also, to put this in perspective, for children and adults alike, not all relationship breakdowns and violations are traumatic. It all depends upon how devastating the situation is to you, the stability of your mental health, previous history of trauma, and the extent of your support system.

When trauma does break your heart, it is apt to close or tighten, in a self-protective move. Inevitably then, healing involves opening again to the warmth of love. Practicing compassion in an intentional way opens the doors that let love in and grief out. So whether trauma occurred recently or many years ago, you can heal—and healing involves learning to be compassionate with yourself.

Your heart is the place of emotional-spiritual healing. In the yoga tradition, the heart area is symbolized by an emerald lotus flower containing a six-pointed star made of a downward-facing and an upward-facing triangle. To see this in your mind's eye, imagine a glowing flower-shaped emerald that holds the Star of David. The triangle pointing down represents compassion and Universal love. The triangle pointing up represents basic human instinctual needs for safety, sexual functioning, power, and self-esteem.

Emotional trauma is a wound to one or more of these basic human instinctual needs. For example, rape can violate personal safety, result in impaired sexual functioning, causing the self-esteem of the rape victim to nosedive into a sense of self as dirty; it's also a betrayal of a woman or man's personal right of choice. Having these basic needs recognized and honored is central to well-being, which is why great emotional pain results when they are violated. This pain takes the form of confusion, anger, fear, grief, and other emotions.

Your heart area is the place where painful emotions related to trauma are healed. Here, mercy and compassion transform emotional wounds into wisdom and emotional strength. Practicing compassion opens your heart and helps you become aware of its warm tenderness. Although this takes some time, your heart can overflow with loving kindness again. When it does, the emotional wounds of trauma are felt, but felt in a new way. Anger becomes grief. Fear becomes understanding. Grief becomes compassion.

You know you are well on your healing way when you can access compassion when you need it. You become able to call upon compassion as a result of doing the compassionate practices taught in the second half of this chapter. In addition to emotional healing there is another result of practicing compassion. You become increasingly less able to be intentionally cruel toward yourself and others. You learn that we are all expressions of Universal love and,

7

in essence, non-separate from one another. That is the most profound healing of all.

So be encouraged, for although you may not be aware of it for some time, each compassionate practice you do touches into loving heart energy. Awaken this love and your heart becomes a place where, no matter what is going on, you can seek shelter and be cared for. Imagine having a shining emerald temple in your heart where you know you are loved. In trauma recovery, learning to feel loved inside is necessary so that facing the wounds of trauma results in healing and not re-traumatization. Treating yourself with reverence allows pain to be seen, felt, and dissolved by the warmth of compassion. Your loving heart, once opened, dissipates your pain, ever so gently, the way the sun melts icicles.

Your healing may be multifaceted, including medical treatment and counseling, yet all along the way you can be compassionate with yourself. Also, if you are currently in external circumstances in which you are not physically safe, the first priority is to get to a safe environment. Doing so is a profound act of compassion. Do not keep your vulnerability a secret. Talk with friends, family, clergy, and law enforcement officers. Find resources to help. Physical safety is first.

The Elements of Compassion

So that you can appreciate the power of compassion, we examine the four elements of compassion.

The First Element: Awareness of Suffering

Compassion cannot arise unless there is awareness of the suffering. Let's look at a real example of suffering being acknowledged.

Marsha, a young schoolteacher, called her mother for comfort one night after a scary episode with her drunken fiancé that resulted in her receiving treatment in a hospital emergency room. The mother, upon hearing her daughter sobbing on the phone, asked, "Oh, sweetheart, what is wrong?" In response, Marsha collapsed into a chair and cried even more, shedding tears of grief and emotional pain. Her suffering, met with kind recognition, began to be released.

Suffering needs to be witnessed, looked at, and admitted to. Otherwise it cannot be openly addressed. When suffering is minimized or shamed, it doesn't go away; it goes underground. If prior efforts to seek comfort from her parents had resulted in dismissal or scolding, Marsha might not have called home for consolation. She might have called a friend or she might not have sought support from anyone. Shame or not believing anyone is there for her may have motivated her to stuff this trauma into a secret. While this response is understandable, keeping her trauma a secret would have robbed her of sharing the pain and receiving compassion. Emotional pain, unseen and not soothed, does not go away—it goes beneath the surface, into body and mind, until it can be released.

The hurts and traumas accumulated in life live on. Fortunately, that which seems unbearable becomes bearable when given loving attention. The bottom line is that it is profoundly healing to have your hurt seen by someone who loves you, and since you are someone who can love you, there is always a person available to you. The point is that you can learn to be there for yourself in increasingly compassionate ways. Plus, if you practice kindness to yourself, before long you will feel safe enough to let others be there for you as well.

Compassion begins with admitting suffering. Begin by simply saying, "I hurt." This simple statement is enough for now. Later in this chapter we teach compassion practices so that you can lovingly tend to hurt.

The Second Element: Recognizing the Sacred Nature of the One Who Is Suffering

The second element is recognizing the sacred nature of the one who is suffering. Marsha's mother's heart felt crushed when she heard Marsha sobbing on the phone, because it was her beloved daughter who was hurt. Compassion is only possible when you realize that you (just like everyone else) are worthy, just because. Practicing compassion to yourself depends upon you becoming like Marsha's mother, so that you look at your pain through the heart of love. David Konstan (2001) says that Aristotle believed that a person cannot have true pity without having gone through suffering of a similar nature, because pity arises from shared experience. Well, you deserve true pity, and you know what you went through. We are social creatures and need others, but we also need to be able to be there for ourselves.

It is crucial to look at your suffering through eyes that appreciate underlying human dignity rather than through eyes that are indifferent. To underscore this point, we turn to the words of Bessel van der Kolk, medical director of The Trauma Center at the Justice Resource Institute in Brookline, Massachusetts. In a webcast filmed at his office on November 22, 2010, titled "Neuroscience and Trauma Theory," he asserted that the most pervasive and damaging type of childhood trauma is not being a delight to your parents. He stated, "Every child needs to light up the room for someone." Louis Cozolino (2010, 206) wrote, "When children are traumatized, abused, or neglected, they are taught that they are not among the chosen." "Not among the chosen" are telling words. Believing that you are not chosen is a big blow. And, as documented by Brian Kolodiejchuk (2007), Mother Teresa poignantly and clearly recognized that being lonely and forgotten transcends age and economic status. For children and adults, not feeling wanted is a fundamental trauma wound.

Healing depends upon you treating yourself with love and dignity. Remember, by its nature, emotional trauma erodes trust and often defiles self-worth. The true cure is in the felt experience of cherishing yourself and life again, no matter what did and did not happen, no matter if the trauma happened when you were a child or an adult. So treat yourself with compassion, even reverence. If you feel tainted and doubting, it is okay—you can still practice compassion. Kindly accept where you are at. Begin with a vow of fidelity: "I know what happened, I am sorry it happened, and I am here for you."

The experience of having someone look at your pain through loving eyes is healing. Some years later, Marsha commented, "My mother knew that my first husband was not good for me, and she still loved me." Marsha was poignantly aware that even though her mother knew about her husband's mistreatment of her, she loved her and did not consider her to be damaged goods. Looking back, she realized that her mother's faithful support was the backbone strength that enabled her to get a divorce. Now, if there was no one there for you, reading this example can activate great yearning. Bear with us, for we teach you how to give yourself the healing compassion you so deserve. We say it again: you can be there for yourself, and you can enlist the most powerful love of all—Universal love.

The Third Element: Understanding

The third element of compassion is understanding. Compassion sees through eyes that appreciate not only how precious human life is but also how impacted we are by violence and mistreatment. In the yoga tradition, the heart is not only the place of compassion, it is also the place of vulnerability. We are innately sensitive, which accounts for the closing of the heart, at least to some degree, when hurt is too great.

Appreciating human vulnerability goes a long way toward alleviating self-blame. In other words, you are not to blame for feelings of confusion, betrayal, distrust, fear, sadness, or rage—or any other emotions. You are sensitive by nature, and having emotions is part of the human experience. You can feel and learn to tend to emotions without labeling yourself as faulty. Likewise, you are not to blame for deficits in relationship skills, emotional-regulation skills, or career-training or life-management skills. Skills are learned, and you can learn, given opportunity.

This understanding allows you to more comfortably accept rather than shun emotions and take steps to learn rather than avoid the effort involved in cultivating skills.

The Fourth Element: Taking Action

The fourth element is taking action. *Karuna*, a Pali word connoting compassion, speaks clearly about action. According to B. K. S. Iyengar (1979, 522), *karuna* is defined as "compassion, pity, tenderness, [and] also implies devoted action to alleviate the suffering of the afflicted ones." Feeling empathy and having sympathetic thoughts are what they are: emotions and thoughts. But compassion takes an important additional step: it takes action. Marsha's mother *acted* compassionately. She demonstrated to Marsha that she was there for her by staying in close contact and gently reminding her that she was a lovely woman who deserved to be treated with love and respect.

We witnessed a woman take compassionate action with her seven-year-old girl during a lunch hour while on retreat with several hundred people. We were in line behind the mother and daughter at the buffet line. The cafeteria was wonderfully quiet, as we were all practicing noble silence and therefore not talking—that is, until this young girl lifted her tray up to place it on the serving rack. The tray tilted and her plate crashed down on the cement floor, noisily breaking into many pieces. Startled by the clamor, people stopped and looked in the direction of this little girl. The girl froze, then wailed loudly and rushed to her mother. Being so young, she was unable to regulate her emotions and needed her mother's assistance. Screaming, she clutched her mother's leg. The woman held her daughter, soothed her with *there, there; you're okay. It was just an accident*, and in a couple of minutes the child's distress subsided. The mother *did* something. She snuggled the girl close to her body and spoke reassuringly. The mother's compassionate action stabilized the girl and imprinted into her daughter some capacity to comfort herself in times of distress.

Compassion as Relationship

Compassion occurs in relationship, between someone who is suffering and someone who extends kindness. Most of us learn how to be compassionate by being the recipient of someone's kindness. Someone responds to our distress in a way that lessens our suffering. It is the kind of response that our friend Jane, a woman with a significant trauma history, described: "I think the kindest thing anyone ever told me was, 'You are enough.' At the end of a session, while saying good-bye, my therapist grabbed my shoulders, looked me in the eye, and said these words to me. I had negotiated so much of myself in trying to please my parents that I was lost and miserable. She helped me see that no matter what I did, it would *never* be enough in their eyes. I collapsed in her arms and cried. My journey of inner peace began that day."

Compassion arises in response to seeing suffering and wanting to do something about it. Clearly, Jane's therapist wanted to do something. Her desire, along with her understanding, prompted her to say the words that Jane had long needed to hear. It was a powerful moment, one that began to free Jane from the anguish of believing that she was not good enough.

Compassionate Relationship with Yourself

You are much more than your traumas, and you are more than a victim. When you totally identify with past difficulties, you become entrenched in them and there is no healing. When you give tender loving care to yourself when the painful thoughts and emotions of trauma arise, rather than collapsing into unhealed trauma, you take care of yourself in a way that allows trauma residuals to be released. Christopher Germer (2009, 89) writes that to "cherish yourself in the midst of pain" is the true meaning of self-compassion. Over time Jane learned to be as tender to herself as her therapist was to her in that great healing moment. She became able to witness rather than cave into upsetting thoughts and emotions and soothe herself by saying, "Sweetheart, remember, you are enough."

When a child you love is hurt, and you know about it, you do your best to help him or her. You certainly do not shame or criticize the child. Aware that you are in a position to offer relief, you do what you can to alleviate his or her distress. Self-compassion is treating yourself with the same loving kindness that you extend to a beloved child.

Once you see or experience compassion, you have a role model for how to be compassionate with yourself. Most people, given the chance to reflect, can remember times when people or animals were compassionate to them. Your primary compassion giver (or givers) when you were young may have been a parent, aunt, teacher, pet, or friend; as an adult it could be those special few in your inner circle or someone who came into your life in an unexpected way. When Rick was young, one of his dearest givers of compassion was his aunt Ruth. "She always welcomed me to her home," describes Rick. "I felt loved by her and safe to be myself. I knew she wouldn't tease me, which was mighty healing since I was often ridiculed."

You deserve compassion—everybody does. The Dalai Lama has often said that no one deserves compassion more than you. No one can give you compassion as reliably as you, since a loved one is not always available when discomfort arises. You are always with yourself and you can learn to take care of fear, loneliness, and pain, even at the most inconvenient times, such as during the middle of the night. When you feel overwhelmed, much like the little girl who dropped her plate, you can learn to soothe yourself, much like the girl's mother did, as long as you remember that you are more than your suffering.

One way to envision how to be compassionate with yourself is by learning from those who treated you with compassion. Experiences of compassion live on in memory, and recalling personal stories of receiving compassion reminds you of the power of compassion and shows you how to be compassionate with yourself.

In calling to mind memories of compassion, look for compassionate actions that are simple and sweet and not directly related to trauma. This lets the learning be tender and not too evocative. Mary offers one memory as an example: "I am directionally impaired and had historically avoided traveling long distances alone. Rick accompanied me on my first seminar tour and offered to come along on my second trip. However, when he informed me that he had to cancel due to a work conflict, I literally collapsed on the office floor in intense fear. I believed that I could not navigate through airports, to rental car offices, and to hotels on my own. Rick waited until my sobbing subsided, then took my hands, looked directly in my eyes, and firmly said, 'You can do this!' His words still stick in my mind. Even though I occasionally get turned around, I *can* travel alone."

Remembering Rick's compassionate response is soothing for Mary. "Bringing to mind how reassuring he was, I feel grateful and emotionally close to Rick," says Mary. "I even feel a little grief, recalling not only how much fear has limited me but how I collapsed into being overwhelmed, unable to witness my thoughts and take care of my fear that evening. I'm also amazed that I can travel by myself." Mary's gratitude arises from feeling cared about and also from the imprinting of the words "you can do it." Those words, now embedded in her mind as a compassionate mantra that Mary repeats to herself, prevent her from falling under the spell of the belief that she cannot learn new skills.

Compassion empowers, and this is important, especially since trauma disempowers, at least for a while. Mary, feeling steadied by Rick's words, flew to Portland, Oregon, navigated a major snow storm, asked for help when she was lost, and discovered that the belief "I can't" was not true. Jane, armed with the words "you are enough," felt empowered to take yoga classes and sign up for meditation retreats. Several retreats later, after learning to sit with herself in silence, she uncovered a profound inner stillness and spiritual connection that gives her great joy and continued healing.

AN INQUIRY INTO MEMORIES OF COMPASSION

As a way to learn to be compassionate with yourself, recall a memory of someone being kind to you. Keep it simple, such as a time when someone offered a helping hand or said reassuring words.

If no one comes to mind think of a pet who jumped on your lap, a song that touched your heart, or the words of spiritual text that were just what you needed to hear at the time. Write about your memory of compassion in your journal, if you keep one.

How does accessing the memory affect you? You may experience tender feelings, just as Mary did. Give yourself a few moments to reflect on how you feel or write about it in your journal.

How were you empowered by this experience of compassion? Pause and contemplate the question and then write about it in your journal if you choose.

Compassion and Your Brain

Compassion is a practice well worth learning because the effects are so profound and even permeate your brain. Compassion does require intentionality, but it is readily available. Kind words are as close as your own mouth, and kind touch is as close as your own hand. All it takes for you and your brain to respond to compassion is simple touch, like placing your hand over your heart or speaking kind words, like the reassuring whisper, "It's okay—relax."

In brief, here is how compassion affects your brain. Soothing words and touch give you something calming to focus on, which, in turn, causes negative and fear-producing thoughts to recede into the background. In the moment of distress, this alone is a great achievement. However, compassion takes it a step further. It strengthens your brain in ways that decreases fear, increases the ability to think clearly, and grows the capacity to view the universe as benevolent.

The human brain is complex, with many parts working together and influencing each other. The compassion circuit consists of more than what can be discussed in this book, but to deepen your appreciation of the power of practicing self-compassion, we highlight a specific part of the brain and its relationship with other brain regions.

The Functioning of the Anterior Cingulate Cortex

One part of your brain cortex, the *anterior cingulate* is notably impacted by thoughts and prayers of compassion. First, consider where it is located, which helps explain its function within the brain. The anterior cingulate sits between the limbic system and frontal lobes. In brief, your limbic system includes the *amygdala*, the part of the brain responsible for keeping you safe. The amygdala scans the environment for threat and when it senses possible danger, your nervous system's emergency fight-or-flight response is activated. Sometimes called the *emotional brain*, it sits in the middle of the brain and is associated with anxiety and anger. The frontal lobe, the brain area above your eyebrows, is called the *thinking brain* and is associated with logic, reason, and language. This is where you assess information, objectively evaluate the external world, and make decisions.

The limbic system and frontal lobes dramatically influence each other. Their relationship is like a teeter-totter—when one side is up, the other is down. When the limbic system revs up, it requires more blood flow, leaving less blood available to flow in the frontal lobes, rendering them less effective. That is why when you are really frightened you can't think clearly. Likewise, when you really focus on reassuring thoughts, the limbic system becomes less active and you feel calmer.

Both are essential to well-being, but they do require a stabilizing force between them, which is the anterior cingulate. It sits between the two and helps to balance emotions and thoughts. According to neuroscientist Andrew Newberg (2009), the anterior cingulate acts like a fulcrum. Like a strong father, it balances the teeter-totter that reason and emotion ride on. In effect, the anterior cingulate dampens fear so that you can reason. It assists with emotional self-regulation and the ability to focus and even recognize errors in reasoning. In other words, activating the anterior cingulate helps you make decisions based on deeper desires than instinctual motivations to be safe, taken care of, and in control. It helps you to take care of fear rather than be dominated by fear in your decision making. This is so important, because fear dramatically reduces options by increasing "I can't" and "It won't work" thoughts, along with many other limiting ideas.

Newberg claims that the anterior cingulate integrates activity within the brain that allows you to see yourself and your relationship with the world more realistically. This is very helpful in correcting the perspective that life is largely dangerous and unsupportive—a view often associated with trauma. In truth, the world is as the world is. You relate to life according to how you perceive it. See life as mostly terrifying and you as its victim, and you respond in ways that attempt to prevent you from feeling overwhelmed. You may avoid feared activities, seek a lifestyle that is secure and predictable, and/or attempt to control others so that you feel powerful and safe. View life as benevolent and yourself as capable of learning and deserving to live, and you have many more options.

Recognizing trauma-based cognitive distortions is step one. Step two is taking action to correct these views. Newberg's research shows that meditating on compassion alters perspective and does so without too much effort on your behalf. On page 126, he states, "It's quite easy to do. Simply focus on compassion or an image of peace as you breathe deeply and relax. Hold this thought for at least twelve minutes a day, and in a matter of a few months you'll begin to build and strengthen new neural circuits of compassion." In this respect, healing is uncomplicated and painless. Simply immerse yourself in memories, words, or images that you associate with kindness and love.

Following are a few examples of how to surround yourself with words that invoke compassion. Rick has the word "kindness" written on a small bulletin board that hangs on the wall to the side of his desk. Mary has the scripture "be still and know" framed and hung on the wall in front of her desk. They are in plain view as consistent reminders.

Jane, the woman whose therapist told her she was enough, has meditated daily for some time using the compassionate words "Let it be" as a mantra. She has recited this phrase often enough that it has taken root in her consciousness, so much so that at times she hears the words, as if they are being spoken to her, from deep within. These stabilizing words are usually easy for her to access when needed, which for her is when she feels stressed, especially about things going on within her extended family. When she starts to feel overwhelmed, she whispers, "Let it be," which allows her to pause, breathe deeply, and regroup.

It takes a little intention and daily practice but, like Jane, you can activate the anterior cingulate and your compassion circuits. It is wonderfully easy. Focus on your favorite compassionate phrase for a few minutes daily. With frequent repetition, the words take up residence in your mind and then the benefits increase. Not only are you soothed during the moments of practicing, after a couple of months you discover that you are calmer and the intensity of old anxieties lessens.

Remember: what you focus on becomes stronger. You already know the power of frightening thoughts. You are probably familiar with the pain of feeling unsupported. It is time to utilize the power of compassionate thoughts. Let's say you frequently think, "I cannot do this by myself." You might therefore post the following words on your bathroom mirror: "You have all the help you need." Whisper those words to yourself whenever you see them and, before you know it, you will hear the echo of those words in your mind, much like the voice of a reassuring friend; you'll find that you can ask for help and accept help when it is offered by others. Mostly though, you are likely to discover that you do not feel so all alone.

SELECT A COMPASSIONATE PHRASE

Search out an inspirational quote on compassion or select a brief scripture. Alternatively, create a phrase that resonates with you. Make it personal; this is for you and doesn't have to make sense to anybody else. Following are three phrases that have deeply personal meaning to the people who chose them.

- "Breathe in kindness, breathe out love."

- "Rest in God's care."

- "Trust, my darling, trust."

Write down your chosen phrase, possibly frame it, and then place it where you will see it.

Meditating on Compassion

When you meditate on compassion you begin to identify more with the desire and capacity to alleviate suffering and less with suffering itself, so that although you experience suffering, you recognize that it is something that happens, not who you are. According to yoga, you are a compassionate being, and your task is to become aware of this fundamental truth. So if you want to truly know yourself, faithfully meditate on compassion.

Two simple practices involve focusing on your heart and paying attention to the sensations and emotions that arise from your chest area. One practice, according to Swami Durgananda (2002) is to focus on breathing into and out from your heart as a simple meditation. Another practice is to place your hands over the chest area and bow to your heart as an act of reverence.

An alternative approach is to meditate on compassionate ideas. Meditating on compassionate ideas is a form of mind training that helps you to approach rather than avoid suffering, teaches you to respond to suffering with kindness, shows you that you are more than your suffering, and cultivates your capacity to extend compassion to yourself and others. As Sharon Begley (2007) reported, this type of meditation is a primary form of mental training for monks, yogis, and other practitioners.

Compassion prayers may be recited by yoga practitioners as a form of meditation. One compassion prayer from the Buddhist tradition, called *Metta* Prayer, helps you to feel deep and abiding empathy for yourself and others.

PRACTICING **METTA** PRAYER

Find a quiet, comfortable place to sit. Settle into your body. Literally feel your feet on the floor and your hips sitting in the chair or meditation cushion. Be aware that you are in your physical body. You may like to place your hand over your heart for a moment as a way to connect with your inner self. Then rest your hands on your lap. Next, with the motivation to generate well wishes and kindness, begin reciting your prayer. Experiment with silently reciting it and then speaking it out loud, and continue with the form that most suits you.

There are several versions of **Metta** Prayer. Here is one form that you may choose to recite:

- May I be peaceful

- May I be happy

- May I be safe

- May I awaken to the light of my true nature

- May [name of person] be peaceful

- May [name of person] be happy

- May [name of person] be safe

- May [name of person] awaken to the light of his or her true nature.

Make the prayer real for you. Start with yourself. For some weeks you may simply recite the prayer for yourself. Then focus on specific people, beginning with loved ones. Gradually add people you feel neutral about, such as the neighbor down the road. Later on, as you are ready, add people you have difficulty with or feel hurt by.

If you find it uncomfortable to wish yourself well, begin the prayer by focusing on someone very dear to you, like a grandchild, but do be sure to include yourself. Even if you do not feel worthy, you yearn for peace. Be gentle, be patient, be persistent, and stay faithful to the meditation. It takes only a few minutes, but you do have to practice, day after day, over a period of time for the prayer to be embedded in your mind. In the meanwhile, with each practice, you have the benefit of connecting in a heartfelt way with yourself and others.

Compassionate Letters to Yourself

Writing compassionate letters to yourself is not a formal yoga practice. However, kindness, so central to healing and yoga, can be accessed in many ways. Compassionate letter writing is a powerful practice that is easy to do. Plus, compassionate letter writing is familiar. If you have written or e-mailed a message of encouragement to someone going through a difficult time, you have written a compassionate letter; and if you have received a note of support during a time of need, you have received a compassionate letter. In both giving and receiving, you felt connected to the other person in a heartfelt way. In a similar manner, you can write and read compassionate letters to yourself that connect the compassionate you to the hurting you.

There is even research that speaks to the healing power of writing compassionate letters to yourself. Paul Gilbert (2010) studied the therapeutic benefits of this form of letter writing in prison settings among inmates, a group of people who has not only caused suffering but also endured suffering. (According to Abram et al. [2004], the majority of inmates have histories of multiple traumas.) The results of Gilbert's work are promising and speak to the central role of compassion in healing trauma.

Gilbert outlines three components of a compassionate letter: understanding, engaging rather than shunning painful feelings, and guidance. The first part of the letter conveys understanding, which allows emotional suffering to be seen, and begins with the words "I understand. ..." The second part of the letter conveys empathy and begins with the words "I know that you feel. ..." The third part of the letter offers guidance to alleviate suffering and begins with the words "My guidance to you is. ..."

Here are examples that may generate ideas about writing your own. First is a letter Mary wrote prior to giving a presentation before an audience of mental health professionals. (Both of us have suffered from fear of public speaking and had panic attacks that either prevented us from giving speeches or made the experience extremely uncomfortable.) "I wanted to be genuine and relaxed with my colleagues," explains Mary, in an effort to contextualize the letter. "Under stress I can fall back into believing that I am not good enough, which causes me to feel tense and try too hard. As a way to introduce compassionate letter writing to the group, I planned to share an example. It dawned on me that if I read a compassionate letter to myself in front of my peers, I would receive a dosage of compassion and also be authentic with them. Following is the letter I wrote and read during the speech."

My dear Mary,

I understand that you fear showing vulnerability, really exposing, and not pretending.

I know that showing vulnerability makes you feel anxious and embarrassed and even ashamed.

My guidance to you is this: You are precious to me. You don't have to be perfectly put together. Your humanness connects you to others. So breathe, my dear, smile, and relax.

While reading the letter to her audience Mary felt transparent and very connected with them. It was a wonderful experience for her.

Rick mentally wrote the following letter while waiting to speak at his father's memorial service. "My father died suddenly and unexpectedly," explains Rick, offering some background, "and the days leading up to his memorial service were very emotional. I have emotionally frozen a couple of times in the past when giving a speech and I didn't want to this time. However, I felt anxious, concerned that I might. While sitting in the pew waiting to read my notes, I heard these words in my head."

Dear Rick,

I understand that you have had difficulty speaking in front of others. I know that you get scared. It's okay. But hear my words: "You are not going to get scared this time. Not this time."

The words "not this time" echoed in Rick's mind, steadying him. When it was his turn to speak to kinfolk and other mourners, he read his prepared words slowly and lovingly.

WRITE A COMPASSIONATE LETTER TO YOURSELF

Write a compassionate letter to yourself. To give it structure, write three paragraphs. Begin the first paragraph with the words "I understand that. ..." In this paragraph write about the situation and your insights into the situation. Begin the second paragraph with the words "I know that you feel. ..." In this paragraph write about your emotional experience. Begin the third paragraph with the words "My guidance to you is. ..." In this paragraph give guidance to yourself.

We encourage you to write a couple more letters. In doing so, you are offering emotional support, acknowledging tender emotions, and giving sage advice.

Embedding Kind Words into Your Physical Body

Words strongly affect your physical body, as you well know. There is that stomach-sinking feeling of hearing about a loved one's health crisis and the heart-melting feeling of a stranger calling to say that he found your lost pet. You may also remember how you felt when someone you were really attracted to said the words "I love you" for the first time. Since words dramatically affect you physically, you can literally massage the words you yearn to hear into your flesh as an intentional compassionate practice. Below is an outline and discussion of this three-part practice.

First: Ask Two Questions

The following two questions are central to the practice:
What do I need to remember?
What do I need to hear?

When Jane, the woman whose therapist told her that she was enough, asked, "What do I need to remember?" she consistently responded with some variation of these two answers: "I deserve happiness" and "You deserve happiness." Both were right on target for her. When she said "I," she affirmed herself as a valuable human being. When she said "you," she reassured the part of her who had ached for fifty years to hear that she was lovable.

Asking the questions matters as much as hearing the answers, since asking conveys loving regard and respect. A clear answer may or may not come. When you ask, you may not hear any answer at all, at least for some time. No answer coming to mind may reflect that you are not used to being asked these kinds of questions. There is not just one answer, and your response may well change over time, so be relaxed with this process. It can take time to open this communication. After experience with this practice, answers do come. If, after reading this discussion, you hear no response when you ask the questions, adopt the words "I am practicing loving kindness to myself." Like most others, you probably benefit from reminders to practice compassion, and with these words you can comfortably continue on with the practice.

Second: Explore a Gentle Massage

The second part of the practice is exploring three partial-body massages. Begin by sitting comfortably with both feet on the floor. With your hands, massage both legs, from your thighs to your ankles. This is a loving massage, so be as sensitive as you are when petting a puppy. Continue for a minute or so. Next, massage each arm with your opposite hand, smoothly stroking upper and lower arms, from your shoulders to your wrists. Next, using both hands, massage the sides of your face, starting with your forehead and moving down each side toward your neck, pausing to give an extra rub to your temples and jawbone. Finally, select the massage that feels most soothing to you and continue on with the practice.

Third: Combine Massage and Recitation

This practice combines a gentle massage and reciting the words that you need to hear. It's as if you knead the words into your skin and muscles. Ideally, speak out loud so that you also hear the words. Repeat the phrase at least five times so that the meaning of the words is taken into your flesh. Jane utilizes this practice as part of her bedtime ritual. It is the last thing she does before covering up. Sitting on the side of the bed, she puts lotion on her legs, then massages her legs, and whispers "you deserve happiness."

This simple, loving, and beneficial technique can be practiced anytime. Give yourself a few minutes of alone time when you do not feel rushed. Sit in a comfortable chair. Ask yourself the two questions, listen for the words you need to remember, choose a simple massage, and recite the words out loud a few times while doing a gentle massage. Give yourself a few moments to feel the effects of the practice. After some experimentation you may find, like Jane did, that you need to hear the same words day after day and that you no longer need to routinely ask the questions. Or you may find that asking the questions is central to your practice.

Compassionate Perspective

Practice compassion and, over time, the footprints of trauma are rinsed out of your body and mind, without you being washed away. No matter how you currently feel or what you believe, you can practice self-compassion. In fact, the part of you that feels wounded may not feel deserving. Understandably, the part of you who yearns to be seen as precious, who desperately needs compassion, may be uncomfortable taking it in for some time. Do not give up on yourself. Your discomfort does not mean that compassion isn't sinking in, but it may take time and consistency in order for traumatized parts of you to begin to trust your motives. Remember, you are more than trauma, more than victim. Compassion is relational and self-compassion comes from outside of the wounded you, from the part of you who desires to do something to help you feel better.

Summary

Compassionate practices infuse the warmth of love and wisdom into the wounds of trauma. You can learn to be compassionate with yourself. Understanding what compassion consists of prepares you for the practices of compassion and helps you appreciate their healing power. The four elements of compassion are: recognizing suffering; realizing that the one suffering, including yourself, is a sacred being; understanding human vulnerability and the effects of trauma; and taking compassionate action.

Practices of self-compassion are powerful acts of compassion that contain the elements of compassion. The practices of compassion taught in this chapter are: inquiring into memories of compassion, reciting compassionate words, meditating on compassion, writing compassionate letters, and embedding kind words with a gentle massage.

chapter 2

trauma, thoughts, and healing

In this chapter we discuss relating to thoughts, including the ideas that you have about the kind of person you are. We review the impact that maltreatment has on self-identity so that you have a clearer understanding of how trauma contributes to self-concept. That knowledge alone is healing, but then we equip you with practices and insights so that you can wisely tend to your thoughts. Throughout the chapter we state that thoughts, which exist outside of your inner essence, are only one small part of the totality of who you are. To begin, we offer a little perspective.

Ongoing emotional trauma can be a form of encoding or internal programming about who you think you are as an individual. The way people who are influential to you speak and treat you dramatically affects your attitudes about yourself. These attitudes coalesce into ideas that influence your self-concept. Self-concept, or your definition of who you are, then generates thoughts in the form of inner voices that make comments such as, "I'm the kind of person who _____." Even though the process of coming up with a self-concept occurs during your developmental years, significant trauma as an adult can modify your sense of who you are.

The yoga philosophy states that you cannot be reduced to your thoughts because fundamentally you are not ideas or beliefs—your own or anyone else's. Yoga teaches you to understand how your mind works, how to relate to attitudes and beliefs, and how to release the grip of the story of self-concept. The truth is that you can learn to have a wise, grandmotherly relationship to these internal voices and thoughts and be relieved of the suffering they cause.

Human Life, Including Yours, Is Sacred

A fundamental message of yoga is that human life is truly sacred. In Pandit Rajmani Tigunait's words (2011, 38), "Yoga's fundamental premise is that to be born as a human is a blessing." This means that you are a sacred being and nothing that happens to you at any stage of your life—and no thought that you think—alters this core truth, including whether or not you feel worthy or believe in higher consciousness. However, when your mind is filled with narratives of unworthiness, the comfort of this truth can be elusive. You may also intellectually understand that you are sacred, yet because you do not feel it in your gut, your life does not feel like a blessing.

It is easy to recognize that you are in the presence of the miraculous when you are around a newborn baby. You somehow know that infant is already worthy, even though unable to do anything to earn self-worth. As a newborn, she or he does not have thoughts about, much less a description of, the kind of person she or he is. Nor is the baby able to look up at you and say, "Hello, sacred being, it is nice to meet my own kind." Self-concept is dependent upon language, the ability to think, and life experiences, all of which take some time to acquire. Like yours, the newborn's sense of identity regarding how lovable and competent she or he is develops during childhood and adolescence. Although it becomes ingrained, it can be influenced, even altered, by primary relationships and significant events throughout life.

One of the keys to healing from trauma is getting to know who you are in the center of your being (that is, interior even to thoughts). You begin to have a dawning sense of your inner self when you confront, even a little, the painful belief that you are unworthy. In fact, during the act of questioning the validity of your *story of me*, also called *false self*, you have a moment of not thinking. That is a precious moment, because when your mind is silent you access the realm of true self, that still place within that is beneath words.

Understanding Your False Sense of Self

Coming up with a story about the kind of person you are is part of human development. Your story may begin with the name your parents gave you at birth. Even though you identify with your name, it is not intrinsic to you. It cannot be, since it is given to you by someone else. In the same way that you adopted your name as an aspect of who you are, you took in the language spoken in your home. You also took in ideas about what men and women are like and a whole lot more. Over time you formulated a self-concept, mostly in the realm of your subconscious mind, by absorbing and reflecting upon life around you. As a result, by the time you were a young adult, you could give an answer when asked to describe yourself. Since significant experiences can alter self-concept, adult trauma can cause a self-concept of being "good enough" to morph into a story of being "damaged."

Yet the yoga philosophy asserts that your story of me, whether it is one of being inferior, superior, or equal, is your false self and not who you truly are! This is because concepts describe your essence as poorly as a blurry photo captures the fullness of the sun rising over mountains. You cannot be reduced to words.

Avidya, a Sanskrit word that means "ignorance" or "darkness," aptly describes your narrative of me. In fact, clinging to the old story of identity keeps you woefully ignorant. In discussing Sutra 8 (about wrong knowledge) from Book 1 of *The Yoga Sutras of Patanjali*, Baba Hari Dass (1999) says that your sense of *I-amness* (arising out of your story) is a form of wrong knowledge that keeps you in a stupor. What a description. Believing your narrative, whether it is positive or negative, keeps you in a daze of false perception. Only when the story of your false self is examined, literally seen for what it is, does your sense of identity expand beyond such limited notions.

Shame-Based Identity

Although self-concept powerfully shapes and limits experiences, everyone has the potential to realize a sense of I-amness that exists beneath the realms of thoughts. Experiencing your own essential goodness is your birthright. However, when your story of me causes too much distress, it takes considerable understanding to see behind it. Yet the veil of ignorance needs to be lifted in order for you to come out of the stupor. Therefore, we offer some insight into a shame-based identity.

Since identity is first formed in childhood, we begin there. Judith Herman (1997, 52) states that "When a parent, who is so much more powerful than a child, nevertheless shows some regard for that child's individuality and dignity, the child feels valued and respected." If you were treated with enough love and respect as a child, you began to sense that you were a worthwhile person. Your story about you was one of being good enough. Having this kind of narrative, even though it falls into the category of false self, does allow you to develop normally.

On the other hand, maltreatment and neglect often create a story of being a damaged self. How could it be otherwise? During the innocence of childhood, you inevitably took in the attitudes and reactions of those you lived with and were dependent upon. How you were and were not protected, cherished, and taken care of entered into your thought processes and eventual sense of identity.

Although we are addressing thoughts in this chapter, we incorporate a discussion on the physiology of shame. Ideas, especially those that pertain to who you are, affect you physically. If you believe that you are a mistake or hear someone whose opinion matters to you say that there is something horribly wrong with you, you are prone to shame, that awful experience of humiliation.

Men, women, children, and adults are vulnerable to the experience of shame. Shame, which first arises in the context of a relationship with someone else, is a normal reaction to being treated in

33

a degrading, oppressive manner. In essence, shame is the inevitable outcome of being dishonored. In Herman's words (1997, 53), "shame is a response to helplessness, the violation of bodily integrity, and the indignity suffered in the eyes of another person." Being humiliated by someone you care about when you are an adult deeply scars your sense of worth; for a child, the experience cuts to the core.

Judith Herman (2007) reports that shame is a "fast-track" physiologic response that comes on quickly and is emotionally painful. A relatively wordless state, shame inhibits speech and thought and causes you to want to hide or evaporate into thin air. Horribly exposing, shame can make you sweat, flush, and feel stupid, as if your utter lack of worth is obvious to anyone in sight, including yourself.

Herman (2007, 12) lists the following vocabulary of shame, which we share to deepen your understanding of how shame shows up mentally and physically: ridiculous, foolish, silly, idiotic, stupid, dumb, humiliated, disrespected, helpless, weak, inept, dependent, small, inferior, unworthy, worthless, trivial, shy, vulnerable, uncomfortable, embarrassed. Truly a body-mind experience, shame feeds into itself. When your body wants to shrink into oblivion, your mind says there must be something shameful about you that needs to be hidden.

If you suffer from a shame-based identity, you innocently slipped behind the veil of a compelling, although false, tale that formed in your mind. Easily triggered, thoughts of worthlessness produce the intolerable sensations of shame. Then, in a state of shame and utter misery, you have little or no breathing space between you and pain-producing thoughts, which is why it is not so easy to come out of the trance of wrong or incorrect knowledge. It's as if you are living an "I'm no good" story line, not just reading the story. Through no fault of your own, you do not know the truth of who you are. Shame and the story of unworthiness interact in a vicious cycle, but one that can be undone.

Self-Inquiry

The healing practices of yoga can help dislodge you from your self-concept, even one as painful as unworthiness. One yoga discipline, called the *study of one's own self*, helps you discern the difference between who it is you merely think you are and who you truly are. Through a process of self-inquiry, you become increasingly aware of the attitudes and beliefs that you have about yourself. While you may already have a pretty clear idea of what you think about yourself, a lot of these thoughts occur in your subconscious mind, where they rumble on, like distant thunder. During inquiry, you first become more aware of the thoughts that so often hang out in the background. Second, you challenge their validity.

The most straightforward inquiry into who you are is the piercing question raised by one of the great yogis of the twenty-first century, Ramana Maharshi. This is the deceptively simple practice of asking the question "Who am I?"

To give you a sense of the practice, here are a few of the hundreds of responses to the question "Who am I?" that we have come up with.

Rick: I am my father's only son, I am the opposite of my father, I am a man, I am from Michigan, I am from Oklahoma, I am stupid, I am smart, I am shy, I am spirit, I am a cat lover, I am my mother's favored son, I am a pilot, I am a consciousness, I am a retreat leader, I am none of the above, I am all of the above, I am caught in a loop, I am tired, I am the wind, I am the witness, I am grateful, I am frustrated, I am hungry, I am a vegetarian. I am—I give up, I do not know!

Mary: I am just a poor girl from Iowa, I am a slow learner, I am a dancer, I am less than I think, I am more than I think, I am a dog lover, I am a homebody, I am a yoga lover, I am a health-food nut, I am silly, I am sensitive, I am bored, I am a walker, I am a reader, I am a counselor, I am okay-looking, I am getting older, I am a spiritual person, I am a mediocre singer, I am goofy, I am peaceful, I am different than I used to be, I am Rick's wife, I am—hmmm, I just know that I am!

SELF-INQUIRY PRACTICE: WHO AM I?

You ask the question, then say your answer out loud or write your answer in a journal. Repeat the question again and again, each time writing or speaking your response. This is a wonderful practice to do regularly, because at the least, it helps you to take your identity story less seriously and expands your sense of self. When you do this inquiry, enjoy the question and be playful with your answers. See how many answers you can come up with. The practice shakes loose your attachment to any fixed notion of who you are and begins to leave you wondering about who you are behind your experiences, circumstances, and thoughts. Also, the practice helps you to realize that you are more than experiences and thoughts, which come and go while you, as awareness, remain constant.

We answered the question with roles, preferences, attitudes, interests, emotions. What we wrote does not point to the essence of who we are any more than what you write reflects your essence, which is interior to concepts. The only constant in the answer to the question "Who am I?" is "I am," which expresses awareness only, not awareness of something. "I am" is a complete description of who you are. This description is sufficient; nothing more is needed, as boggling and unsatisfactory as this may be to your mind.

Ramana Maharshi's teaching was clear and direct. He is quoted (Osborne 1972, 40) as saying, "Pure awareness is what I am." He also suggested not replying to the question "Who am I?" in words. Rather than responding, let the question be unanswered. By letting the mind remain quiet you are aware and alert, yet not thinking.

This is the truest answer to the question because in reality no words can fully describe you.

Although you inevitably and naturally identified with a self-concept, it is a form of false knowledge. Luckily, great possibility awaits you. You do not have to remain confined to that level of understanding. Whatever happened to you happened, what was said was said, and none of that can be undone. Fortunately, nothing has to be undone; something has to be recognized. You are not experiences; you have experiences. You are not roles; you play roles. You are not thoughts; thoughts pass through you. Your healing depends upon you becoming aware of how painfully, albeit inevitably, you identified with circumstances and ideas.

Another beloved Indian guru, Sri Nisargadatta (1990, 375) reports that his guru told him, "You are not what you take yourself to be." He is also quoted as saying, "My Guru ordered (me) to attend to the sense 'I am' and to give attention to nothing else. ... Whatever happened I would turn my attention from it and remain with the sense 'I am.'" Accordingly, his teaching is "*tat tvan asi*," meaning "divinity you are."

The famous Sanskrit mantra "*neti, neti*" translates to "not this, not this." *Neti, neti* is a form of self-inquiry, as it points to the truth of who you are by clearly defining who you are not. An extraordinary mantra, it points to the truth that there is no thought, no story, that fully describes you. Since you are beyond any man- or woman-made story of identity, any word that suggests a shame-based identity is simply, unarguably, not true.

Mary's Experience with Father Thomas Keating

In 1999 Mary interviewed Father Thomas Keating, a Trappist monk who lives in Snowmass, Colorado. During the interview she asked him to talk about low self-worth. He responded with, "Low self-worth is an innocent misunderstanding. It occurs when you do not know who you are, when you do not know that you are your Father's child." Mary began to weep. A veil of ignorance was lifted and she felt some formerly unrecognized aspect of herself rise up from deep within. In being seen by Father Keating, she was able to know herself in a new way. That evening, she experienced a meditative dream that directly addressed Mary's taking herself to be something that she is not. She realized that she is not the product of her circumstances. We include it here because the truth that it revealed about human life being sacred is equally valid for you.

"I was taken on a life review in my dream," says Mary. "It was as if God entered my mind and revisited childhood and early adulthood with me. Together, looking out from my eyes, as one, we saw many scenes. Then I heard very clearly, 'I have always been with you and am with you always.' A profoundly healing experience, it shattered my belief in the story that I was unworthy.

"Since then," Mary continues, "I generally do not believe the story line of being a poor girl from Iowa who is not as good as other people. Occasionally I forget and fall under the spell of the old false identity, which I experience as a shame attack. Feeling wretched is my clue to wake up, and sooner or later I do. As stupefying as shame is, it does send a loud message to come out from behind the unworthiness curtain."

You are "not this, not this" no matter what awful things have happened or how desolate you feel. It is possible that you got covered up with circumstances and became unable to see yourself clearly. Fortunately, you can learn to see yourself through uncontaminated eyes.

Meditation

A fundamental yoga practice, meditation cultivates three capacities that help you to recognize who you are behind thoughts. These three capacities are concentrating, witnessing, and resting in inner stillness. When you develop these skills you are able to relate to thoughts rather than be held captive by them. Concentration helps you to move your attention away from thoughts, witnessing helps you to become aware of the kinds of thoughts your mind generates, and resting in inner stillness makes you aware that you are more than what you think.

Your capacity to relate wisely to your thoughts begins with learning how to focus your attention.

Concentrating Your Mind

Learning to concentrate is central to healing. Here is why. Your attention, unharnessed, is as unpredictable as an untamed stallion. Wild, it goes all over, including to places in your mind that you wish it would not. On the other hand, your attention, well trained, is as powerful as a winged horse. Once you can say, "I am going to focus on this and not that," you can take good care of your thoughts.

Concentration meditation practice, which we present shortly, trains your attention to focus on what you want it to. You know the experience of having thoughts you wish would leave you alone, yet your attention keeps going back to them. It is a miserable experience that debilitates. Luckily, you can train your attention to focus on ideas and sensations (such as breathing) that steady and empower you.

When you divert attention away from thoughts and focus on breath or a sacred mantra, thoughts recede into the background. Attention may drift back to thoughts, but as soon as you realize that your attention is not going in the direction you desire, you can redirect it. This is how you cultivate concentration. Over time, with repeated practice, you can harness your attention as reliably as you can lead a well-trained horse.

Concentration and Your Brain

Concentration is a function of the *prefrontal cortex*, the part of your brain that sits above and behind your eyebrows. This brain region is pliable, meaning it is trainable. A fundamental way to train it is with concentration practices. Each time you intentionally pay attention to your breath (or another object of focus) you strengthen your prefrontal cortex's ability to move your attention away from some thoughts and redirect it toward other thoughts, at will.

In essence, concentration meditation is attentional training because it is a practice of focusing on something specific, on purpose. What you focus on is optional. Breath awareness, gazing at a sacred symbol, and mantra or sacred word recitation are traditional yoga practices, so we present all three. After discussing them we give instructions for meditation.

Breath Awareness Concentration Meditation

There are good reasons to select breath awareness as a focal point for meditation. First of all, breath is always available. Second, focusing on breath directs attention into your body and away from your mind. This quiets your thinking mind. Third, focusing on breath, which is a physical sensation, makes you aware of your body. This is an experience of being centered in body rather than thoughts, which causes you to feel grounded. Experience this for yourself. Pause for a moment and pay attention to an in breath and an out breath. Notice that your mind becomes quiet and you feel grounded.

Breath draws in vital life energy, which keeps you alive and utterly connected to life outside your body. Focusing on breath in meditation can increase your awareness of the life force in which you live and breathe. Interestingly, even language points to the unity of breath and something transcendent. The English word "spirit" comes from the Latin word *spiritus*, which means "breath." The Greek word for "spirit" (*pneuma*) and the Hebrew word for "spirit" (*ruach*) also mean "breath." It is no wonder then that you experience yourself and life joined together as one when your attention is fully absorbed in breath. While you may think that you are disconnected, in reality you are not.

You may also find it natural to close your eyes when focusing on breath. This is a retreat from the outer world. Reducing sensory input shuts out the world of objects, which can increase your awareness of the connection you have with vital life energy.

When actually meditating, once your mind is quiet, there is no need to focus on breathing. Simply sit and enjoy the inner stillness. When attention drifts back toward thoughts, gently return your focus to your breath until silent awareness once again predominates.

Gazing Concentration Meditation

Looking at an object, such as a candle flame, a fresh flower, a sacred symbol, or the picture of a spiritual person, is a soothing meditation. In this meditation you gaze at something that represents the divine as a way to relate, through your eyes, to higher consciousness. This is a soft gaze—there is no need to stare or not blink. At first, you are aware of distance between your eyes and what you are looking at. Then the sense of space dissolves and you become absorbed in or feel at one with the flickering light, orchid, or whatever else you are seeing. It's as if you merge with the object and no longer experience yourself as disconnected from it. Once again, there you are, aware of the oneness of life.

This gentle meditation can feel psychologically safe since your eyes are open and you can see what is going on around you. Also, open eyes help you to remain comfortably alert in meditation and symbolizes awakening to the truth of your sacred nature.

Mantra Concentration Meditation

Mantra meditation consists of quietly chanting a sacred word or phrase over and over and is sometimes referred to as the *prayer of the heart*. In this meditation you literally fill your mind with the sound of the divine by repeating a word or phrase such as "Beloved," "Divine Mother," or "My Lord." At the least, mantra meditation invites relationship with the divine and has the potential of invoking an experience of deep spiritual union.

Within the yoga tradition, a sacred Sanskrit mantra "*So Ham,*" translated as "He is I" or "It is I," is frequently recited in meditation. You may prefer the mantra "I Am," from Psalm 46:10: "Be Still and Know That I Am God," if it is more familiar to you. Another revered Sanskrit chant is "*Shree Ram*" (loosely translated as "radiant embodiment of bliss and salvation"). Two examples of people who practiced mantra meditation are Gandhi, who recited "*Ram,*" and Mother Theresa, who recited the word "God" with her rosary.

In this meditation you silently repeat a selected mantra until you enter into the domain of pure silence. When that happens, simply enjoy being aware of deep peace. There is no need to interrupt pure silence with a mantra. Then, when attention wanders off to thoughts, refocus on your mantra until again experiencing aware silence.

As yoga practices are not a religion and are appropriate for people of many faith traditions, we include a Christian mantra meditation practice called *centering prayer*. Brought into contemporary Christianity by Father Thomas Keating, this practice is defined as a way to open to the presence and action of God in the center of your being. Father Keating (2010) likens this meditation to an act of friendship with God that becomes deep communion. He also emphasizes that God appreciates all your efforts toward friendship. He recommends beginning meditation by silently whispering a sacred term, such as "*Abba*" or "Our Father," to invite and consent to God's presence and action in you. Then sit quietly. When thoughts arise, silently say your chosen sacred word until your mind becomes quiet again. When you enter into stillness, you experience yourself in a pure way that is profoundly healing.

PRACTICING CONCENTRATION MEDITATION

Select breath awareness, gazing at a sacred object, or reciting a mantra as your focal point. Explore all three to find the one that feels most natural or somehow right for you. After some experimentation, stay with one focal point for your sessions rather than switching them out. Also, begin with just a few minutes, if that feels most doable for you. Gradually lengthen your practice, up to twenty minutes or more. Concentration meditation is so valuable that the minutes dedicated are well worth the effort.

Select a time of day to practice, preferably when your household is quiet. Early morning is especially nice, as it sets the tone for the day. Choose a comfortable chair or cushion in a quiet place, one that you are drawn to. Ideally, sit up straight. However, if sitting is uncomfortable, recline in a position that is easy to be in. Practice in a posture that is pleasing and easy to return to most days.

To truly benefit, practice regularly. You do not have to sit for an hour. Research shows that even a twelve-minute practice makes a difference. Andrew Newberg (2009) reported that US senior citizens who recited the Sanskrit mantra "**Sa Ta Na Ma**" (translated as "Infinity, Birth, Death, Rebirth") twelve minutes a day for eight weeks produced positive changes in their brains. Practice concentration meditation to tap into the sacred within and all around you, gain freedom from trauma, and take good care of your brain.

The Inner Experience of Concentration Meditation: Focus, Witness, and Stillness

To describe what the experience of concentration meditation is apt to be like on the inside, we've selected breath awareness as an example. It begins with focus. Sitting comfortably, you begin to pay attention to breathing. Before long, your attention wanders off to what you are thinking. There you are, lost in thought, until you realize what is happening.

As soon as you become aware of your thoughts, you are no longer lost in them. Meditation continues as you witness. As you observe thoughts, just observe—there is no need to do anything with them. Let them be and they pass by like leaves floating in the current of a stream. You may even have a thought of recognition and spontaneously think, "Wait a minute—I am meditating." Witness even that thought, then refocus on breathing, because in meditation witnessing leads to refocusing.

There are moments when all is silent inside. By the way, this is not being zoned out or in a trance, whereby you eventually come to or pop back from a foggy state. Rather than being unaware, you are aware, alert but not thinking, conscious but not focusing when silence overtakes you. There you are, resting in the stillness of your deep interior, which feels incredibly peaceful, safe, and fulfilling. Soon enough, thoughts arise and distract you until you once again become aware of what is happening. Your experience may move from focus to witness to experiencing alert stillness many times in one session.

To further explore the inner experience we turn to Father Thomas Keating (2010), who gives easy-to-remember suggestions for relating to thoughts as they arise. Do not resist, retain, or react to thoughts. Resisting thoughts, an act of aversion, pushes them into subconsciousness. Retaining thoughts, an act of attachment, reinforces them, and reacting to them creates emotional energy.

Simply, nonviolently, let thoughts be and focus on breathing until silence overtakes you. Resting in silence during meditation is the true aim of meditation, and concentrating and witnessing are what quiet your mind.

Understanding and Taking Care of Thoughts

Left to itself, your mind generates thoughts that seem to go all over the place, drifting hither and yon, in a stream of thoughts that scientists call *default network*. The contents of thoughts can be as varied as the movement of the wind. However, in the same way that the wind is limited to the four directions, thoughts are limited to four categories. Swami Rama (1976) reported that, according to the yoga philosophy, the mind produces thoughts that fit into four main categories: the future, the past, the story of me (false sense of self), and judgment or assessment.

Learning to categorize your thoughts helps you to find out which types of thoughts predominate. For instance, you can discover if your thoughts drift more to the future or the past. You can learn how often judgmental thoughts and story of me thoughts arise. To categorize thoughts, simply state to which of the four categories the arising thought belongs. When you hear thoughts that fret about tomorrow, say "future"; when you hear thoughts that despair about the past, say "past." When a thought scolds, such as "What were you thinking? Why did you do that?" say "judgment." When a thought pouts, such as "Things never work out the way I want," say "story of me."

The act of categorizing a thought puts some space between you and it, which diffuses the influence the thought has on you. Literally, in the moment of categorizing a thought, you are no longer emotionally under its spell. Categorizing a thought buys you a couple seconds of quiet that allows you to make an intentional choice. Often it helps to focus on breathing or a mantra for a little bit to quiet your mind even more. This steadies you so that you can deliberately decide what to focus on next to prevent your attention from drifting back to those old familiar thoughts that do not help you.

Imagine being able to respond to the thought "There is something horribly wrong with me" with "story of me." This sounds easy enough, however, in reality it is a daunting task. These old stories have been circulating in your mind for many years and they are not readily dismissed. Some thoughts you have heard well over a thousand times. In fact, when you respond with "story of me," you are likely to hear a rebuttal, something such as "You think you are so smart, categorizing thoughts—well, it won't work." When this happens, gently whisper, "judgment" or "judging critic" (discussed in the next sections) and BREATHE as if your sanity depends on it. Then intentionally get up and get busy doing something constructive, like loading the dishwasher.

You cannot control the thought but you can witness, categorize, and take your attention off of it. Left unattended, the thought drifts away like a leaf in the current of a stream. You, on the other hand, are left alone to make a healthy choice for yourself.

Your Inner Critic

Even the yoga sages of more than two thousand years ago encountered judgmental thoughts. However, it was left to Sigmund Freud, who lived from 1856 to 1939, to coin the term *superego*, which describes the aspect of your mind that tries to trick you into behaving according to some prescribed, ideal way and scolds you for not measuring up. The more recent concept of *inner critic*, popularized this past decade, is very similar to superego. The inner critic refers to an inner voice that attacks your worth. It comes up with thoughts about how bad, wrong, or insufficient you are.

The *judge*, or *gremlin*, as it is popularly named in self-help books, demeans, discourages, and reinforces your sense of self as unworthy.

If you have a shame-based story of identity, it is likely that your inner critic is severe with you, making sure that you do not come out from under the suffering of unworthiness. Unfortunately it can be very harsh, even virulent. As one associate said, "My inner critic has a PhD and knows all the ways I try to escape it or get rid of it." Try as you might, you cannot completely, for once and for all, shut it up.

Relating to Your Inner Critic

It is imperative to steer your attention away from the inner critic so that you are not beaten up by it. Move your attention to something safer, like your breath. Literally back your attention away from the harsh words. Give yourself a moment to breathe and regroup. Whisper "judging critic" and then withdraw your attention from it. Like other thoughts, the harsh words of the inner critic roll on down the stream of thoughts when you redirect your focus onto your breath. If its words come back in the next second, and the second after that, repeatedly place your attention on breathing. To really divert your attention, get up and do something.

There is no one perfect way to relate to your inner critic. You have to find your own way. Whatever you do, first call it by its name, take a deep breath, and do some mundane task. Here is what James, a man who used to frequently collapse into self-loathing, learned to do. "My inner critic's voice is like an unrelenting hammer that pounds on me," described James. Ignoring his inner critic was next to impossible. He said, "I can't ignore being hammered on." Something more was needed. After some experimenting he named the inner critic "You." When necessary, James would raise his hand up in the air, like you do when getting someone's attention, and say, "You, not now." He would say "not now" in the same fatherly, firm voice that he disciplined his young sons with when they were overly rambunctious in public. This response bought him just enough time to redirect his attention to doing some routine chore, like putting fresh water in the dog's water dish.

After about a year of this practice, James no longer had to raise his hand, at least not most of the time. He could let the inner critic's voice (which is a thought, after all) go by like a clump of leaves in a stream. He realized that the voice of the inner critic, like thoughts of racism and sexism, belongs to the category of collective judgmental thoughts. Harsh judgment can come from yourself as well as others. Like other prejudicial attitudes, the voice of the inner critic causes great suffering. "And," James said, "history is filled with painful examples of what happens when some people are categorized as inferior to others."

He recognizes the toll the voice of the inner critic has taken on his esteem and acknowledges that, at times, the punch of the inner critic still takes his breath away. But, thanks to the strength of a daily meditation practice, he is a skilled observer of his inner life, including the inner critic. He recovers from its caustic words more quickly then he used to. As soon as he becomes aware of what is going on, he takes a deep breath and says, "Wait a minute—look at what happened." Then he stands up, literally, and steps out on the deck or gets a drink of water. He understands the voice of his inner critic and knows how to relate to it.

Relating to Your False Self Story

While you cannot be separate from your sacred nature, you can be agonizingly unaware of it. However, you are not who you take yourself to be. Without a shadow of a doubt, the shame or trauma victim story is not who you are.

Relate to your false self story by first recognizing it. Give it a personalized name if you like, something like "little me." Then, when you hear its voice, whisper its name and take a breath. Sometimes that response is sufficient to recover your equanimity. However, the voice of the false self can be associated with a lot of pain. When it is, you may want more of a response. Since the story of me is a case of mistaken identity, after breathing and naming it focus on words that point to your true self. Following are some suggestions.

Whisper "not this, not this" when the false self voice says that you are inferior or superior, for neither is the truth. Alternatively, sing "I Am" as a chant. Sing along to the beautiful melody of "Amazing Grace" or even to the tune of "Happy Birthday to You." Make your chant or song enjoyable and you may find that you feel better immediately.

Here is the bottom line: Your mind is capable of heavenly and hellish thoughts about you, others, and life. That is just the way it is. When you understand how your mind operates and know how to focus, you can be selective about which thoughts you pay attention to. Focus on heavenly ideas rather than hellish thoughts. Singing the refrain "I Am" speaks about your true self. What a heavenly idea.

Buddhi: True Intelligence

The yoga tradition identifies another voice, one that speaks words of great insight. This voice comes from beyond the thinking mind and its four thought categories. This voice, the expression of true intelligence, arises out of silence.

The Sanskrit word for this voice is *buddhi*. Buddhi, the source of wisdom, communicates as inner guidance. You may sense it as a hunch, intuition, or inner knowing. Buddhi tends to arise when your mind is quiet or it may just be that you are more able to hear it then. This is why it is prudent to make significant decisions after quiet reflection. The advice to sleep on important decisions is indeed sound because during sleep your thinking mind quiets down. Then, early the next morning, before your mind gets busy, you are likely to hear the voice of inner guidance. Meditating, which quiets the thinking mind, also makes it easier to hear insights about important matters, including what is needed for healing.

Filling Your Mind with Knowledge of the Sacred

One yoga discipline is studying scriptures. Scriptures teach you about ultimate reality, point you to your spiritual essence, and infuse you with the presence of the divine. Paramhansa Yogananda (1946, 221), a twentieth-century yogi master, states that "no true freedom for man is possible without knowledge of the ultimate Reality." Reading scriptures and reciting the name of God are practices that correct painful, faulty thinking. They embed sacred truth into your mind and confront your identification with your false self story.

Summary

The main message of this chapter is that you are not who you think you are. Although it is normal to formulate a concept of who you are, it is contrived, man-made. Your false self-identity arises and is maintained within the context of life experiences. Significant maltreatment often results in a painful story of unworthiness that is way off track, simply wrong. The things that happened and did not happen to you are experiences that affected you. They are not your identity.

Yoga practices help you to understand your mind so that you can take care of thoughts that cause you anguish. Concentration meditation practices cultivate your ability to concentrate, witness thoughts, and become attuned to profound stillness deep inside. Two of the primary focal points for concentration meditation—

breath awareness and mantra recitation—transfer into skills that help you take care of pain-producing thoughts.

Self-inquiry and learning to categorize thoughts help you to wisely relate to thoughts. Self-inquiry enables you to confront the legitimacy of the false self. Categorizing thoughts puts distance between you and pain-producing thoughts, such as thoughts that judge you harshly. Then, utilizing the skills of concentration, witnessing, and focusing on breath, you can relate to the false self and inner critic in ways that heal and comfort. Mantra recitation and study of the sacred scriptures fills your mind with the knowledge of the blessed nature of life, including yours.

chapter 3

emotional trauma, physiology, and healing

emotional trauma can have a profound and lasting impact on health and happiness. It permeates life experience more deeply and heals more slowly than physical injuries that leave bruises and break bones. Over time bones mend and bruises heal. Yet time alone does not heal emotional trauma, whose wounds are held deep within. Emotional trauma lingers on because of the way it affects the brain and nervous system. This trauma also greatly impacts self-esteem and relationships with others.

Fortunately, you can help heal the wounds of emotional trauma. Understanding emotional trauma and how it affects the brain and nervous system supports recovery. It is easier to help yourself heal when you know what you are dealing with and how to help yourself. In this chapter we describe and define emotional trauma and the ways it affects the nervous system and brain. We then illustrate how gentle yoga breathing practices can help release trauma from your nervous system.

Emotional Trauma

Being personally mistreated or seeing someone else horribly wounded impacts deeply and may make you wonder how such cruelty is possible. And witnessing the death and destruction associated with natural disasters, war, or terrorist attacks can erode your faith in life's goodness. The more closely trauma touches you, such as being at the scene or knowing someone who was hurt, the greater the potential for long-lasting impact. That is why first responders to large disasters and individuals who helplessly witness loved ones being injured are at high risk for experiencing emotional trauma responses. Likewise, if trauma separates you from loved ones or leaves you homeless, you are more vulnerable to the effects of emotional trauma.

As Brian Trapper (2009) reported, psychological well-being requires being in an environment that emotionally nurtures and provides basic needs for food and shelter. Therefore, if your home is destroyed in a natural disaster, your personal trauma is greater than is the neighbor's who loses his garage. Likewise, if you and your children's safety are threatened and you have to hide from your spouse, your risk of emotional trauma is great.

With the exception of physical violence that leaves lasting injury, it is psychological trauma that lives on in your nervous system, long after flesh and bones have healed. For example, if you accidentally tripped on a rug, fell down a flight of steps, and fractured your arm, you would probably heal with little residual physical or emotional damage other than perhaps being cautious when stepping on rugs at the top of steps. If, however, your arm sustained a fracture as a result of being pushed down a flight of steps many years ago by your grandfather or recently by your partner, your arm healed yet you probably have lingering emotional trauma. In this case, it is not the broken arm but the betrayal of trust, the unkind words, and unpredictable violent act of a family member that distressed your nervous system and sense of well-being.

Emotional trauma results when something happens that shatters your sense of safety, your ability to cope, and perhaps even your self-worth. That event can be an acute situation, such as forced sex, or a chronic condition, such as being raised by a mentally unstable parent. Emotional trauma may or may not be connected to physical trauma. Your grandfather or partner threatening to push you down the steps, without actually shoving you, is assault enough to shake your sense of safety, make you fearful, and cause you to feel shame.

Emotional trauma occurs to people of all ages. Everyone, even people with little prior trauma exposure, has a breaking point. No one is immune; however, if you were raised in a stable, loving family you have some protection against the negative effects of trauma. Having people in your life to support you and few instances of previous trauma that can be reactivated does buffer you from the effects of unfortunate events. However, no matter how old you are, human cruelty and natural disaster take a toll.

Childhood Adversity Is Pervasive

Adult trauma is difficult whether or not you experienced trauma when you were growing up. It is also true that trauma occurring during childhood can have pronounced effects on adult functioning and well-being and put you at risk for adult trauma. Take this simple analogy: Anyone can break a bone when falling off a horse; however, the risk for bone fracture is higher and healing takes longer for someone who has osteoporosis, or less-dense bones. Likewise, anyone can be hurt by another's cruel words, however, adult trauma can reactivate old emotional wounds in someone who was verbally battered as a child.

It is helpful to be informed about childhood trauma so you can accurately assess if and how your life has been touched by it. Statistically speaking, if you were raised in the United States, it is quite possible that you have been affected by childhood trauma. More than 50 percent of respondents of a large survey reported that they had experienced adversity in early life, including witnessing parental abuse (Felitti et al. 1998). This sad state of affairs certainly undoes the belief that trauma occurs infrequently.

Emotional trauma can occur without physical violence, yet it is an aspect of physical abuse and, unfortunately, violence is very prevalent in this country. Scan through these staggering statistics on violence in US homes. In December 2011, the National Centers for Disease Control and Prevention reported that one in four women and one in seven men have experienced severe physical violence by an intimate partner at some point in their life. This is devastating for everyone involved, including children, because seeing your parent being mistreated models cruelty, disrespect, and emotional pain as an aspect of intimacy. David Finkelhor (2005) reports that one in three children is exposed to violence, not including what is seen on television and in movies.

The statistics listed in the last paragraph are heartbreaking. However, as we stated, emotional trauma is not limited to witnessing or directly experiencing physical abuse at home. As the following authors indicate, exposure to trauma is the norm, not the exception for children in this country. William Copeland and colleagues (2007) found that two-thirds of children were exposed to one or more traumatic events by age sixteen and, in an extensive national survey, Finkelhor and collaborators (2009) reported that one in five children experiences some form of child abuse or neglect. Childhood trauma is so pervasive in this culture that Bessel van der Kolk (2011), a highly respected trauma researcher and treatment expert, called it a public health problem because of the long-lasting effect it has on physical and mental health.

We want to state that not everyone who experienced adversity in early life ends up with a criminal record, broken relationships, or major health problems. Many people who experienced severe difficulties in childhood have gone on to create loving homes and become contributing members to society. In fact, according to Ronald Kessler (1995) most people (50 to 90 percent) encounter trauma during a lifetime, yet only about 8 percent develop full posttraumatic stress disorder (PTSD, a specific response to trauma that includes chronic states of anxiety and various ways of reexperiencing the trauma, including flashbacks).

Childhood Neglect

The National Child Abuse and Neglect Data System (NCANDS) reports that neglect is by far the most widespread form of childhood maltreatment.

Emotional neglect, not readily seen by outsiders, often accompanies the other forms of neglect, which are categorized as not having safe shelter, adequate food, medical care, or proper schooling. Potentially devastating, emotional neglect of a child consists of failure to provide love, affection, encouragement, and a stable home environment. Emotional neglect can have an insidious impact that cannot be stopped unless identified. Therefore we list the major types of emotional neglect and make them real by adding a personal commentary. If you identify with these experiences, we hope that reading them helps you to feel less alone and more encouraged to stay the course of your healing.

Ignoring

You were ignored if your parents consistently failed to respond to, or disregarded, your needs for love, interaction, and nurturance. As a child you needed to be encouraged and acknowledged as being real and worthy in order to develop healthy self-esteem and feel emotionally connected to others. Catherine, a woman who has overcome significant childhood trauma, described being ignored in these words: "I don't remember being hugged by my mother, even though I know she took care of me before she became so depressed, nor do I recall being greeted when I came home from school. I felt unimportant to [her] in so many ways."

Isolation

If your parents prevented you from having friends or seeing your relatives you probably felt alone and different from others. Children need social contact with others, both adult and children. Oftentimes, children who are isolated are also physically abused. Catherine described it like this: "I was always alone, outside of school. I never (not exaggerating) had a friend over to my house. No relatives dropped by. The silence at home was deafening. I spent most of my time in my bedroom, especially when my father was drinking."

Exposure to Parental Violence

If you heard or saw one of your parents being hit or beaten by your other parent or another adult, or heard loud arguments and other sounds of abuse followed by tears or silence, you were exposed to spousal violence. Catherine continued by saying, "I locked my bedroom door when my parents fought. I don't know what I hated more: my mother's pleas, doors slamming, or the awful silence that followed."

Emotional Abuse and Maltreatment

Emotional abuse is the core of all forms of abuse, whether you are a child or adult. Acts (words) of maltreatment send a painful message, one that says you are worthless, unloved, flawed, or in danger. Emotional abuse linked with emotional neglect is called *emotional maltreatment* (Iwaniec, Larkin, McSherry, 2007). The well-known phrase "Sticks and stones may break my bones, but words will never hurt me" is simply not true. Slaps may bruise your skin, but words are invisible arrows that penetrate heart and mind, no matter your age.

Types of Emotional Abuse

Following is a list of some types of emotional abuse. We include this list in order to educate you about what emotional abuse consists of and also as a way for you to recognize abuse that you have experienced. Again, emotional abuse happens to adults and children. We continue with examples from childhood, as in this chapter we are highlighting early-life maltreatment.

Ridicule

Being criticized or belittled by a parent, spouse, or loved one shakes your sense of self-worth and, when it happens in childhood, ongoing ridicule shapes your sense of identity. Mary heard these words from her grandmother, a tired woman who was embittered by poverty and fatigued from a life of hard work: "Who do you think you are, Miss Fancy Pants? Don't ever forget which side of the tracks you grew up on. You are nobody special, so stop trying to act like you are." Those words stung and sent a message of unworthiness.

Indifference

Being ignored or regarded as not mattering, whether by a boss, siblings, or close associates, can make you feel lower than low, even with a good enough upbringing (meaning your basic needs for food, shelter, medical care, and education were met; you got to be a child; and you were loved and encouraged enough). However, if early-life caretakers were distant or uninvolved, as an adult you may stay in friendships and job environments that are not nurturing because that is what you know. Here is another example from Catherine, who often heard words such as these from her father: "Go away. Just leave me alone. Can't you see that you are bothering me?" Being disregarded in intimate relationships became normal for her.

Rejection

Whether you are a man, woman, teenager, or child, painful and consistent rejection by someone who is supposed to love and care for you sends the message that you are not among the chosen. Phrases such as "I wish you had never been born," "You were a mistake," and "Something is wrong with you" show disregard and contempt for who you are. Even though such damaging words are not at all representative of who you are, an innocent child is apt to take them as truth.

Harassment

Being picked on and bullied can result in you feeling terrified and uncared for, especially when done by someone close to you. You have probably experienced an aggressive driver cutting you off or someone threatening or attempting to intimidate you. No matter how you acted on the outside, inside you most likely felt fear or anger. Being harassed by a stranger is upsetting for an adult, but when it is a family member and you are a child the effect is amplified. Rick recalls this experience: "When I was nine, while helping my father in the garage, he asked me to hold a chisel on a part so that he could hit it with a hammer. I held the chisel, but when he swung the hammer I dropped it, fearing he would miss and hit my hand. My dad asked, 'Are you afraid that I'm going to miss and hit you?' He then grabbed my hand, hit my thumb with the hammer hard enough to hurt and scare me, and said, 'Stop crying and hold the chisel or I will hit your thumb again.'"

The Effects of Trauma on the Brain

Knowing a little about what trauma does to your brain, then later reading about what yoga does to your brain, helps you to understand how yoga heals trauma. This section introduces you to some brain structures that pertain to three crucial areas of functioning: your ability to bond with others, to regulate your emotional ups and downs, and to feel good about who you are. Undeniably, trauma in early life affects your brain and your life. As Louis Cozolino (2010) reported, early life experiences molded your brain in ways that affect the vitally important areas of attachment (emotional bonding, trust, and reliance), emotional regulation (soothing distress), and self-esteem (whether you value yourself as a human being).

In an abbreviated way we are going to outline three main brain structures.

Brain Stem

We begin with the brain-stem region, the part of your brain that governs basic physiological processes. This primitive brain region contains the *autonomic*, or involuntary, nervous system, which governs the actions and functions of organs, including heart, lungs, and digestive tract. This part of your brain is fully developed at birth. We discuss the effect of trauma on the autonomic nervous system in greater detail shortly.

Limbic System

The second brain region, also fully developed at birth, is the *limbic system*. Located in the middle of your brain, this area also has crucial functions that include emotionally bonding with loved ones. Contained within the limbic system is the *amygdala*, whose job it is to scan the environment for danger. Always on the lookout, the amygdala sends out messengers that trigger the fight-flight-freeze response when it senses danger so that you can quickly respond, before you can even think. It can react to a potential threat more than ten times faster than it takes for the same experience to register in your conscious awareness. According to Stefan Wiens (2006, 313), it takes 500 to 600 milliseconds for an experience to register in conscious awareness, while the amygdala can react to a potential threat in less than fifty milliseconds. Responsible for your survival, it remembers all threats, compares incoming data to what is in its memory banks, and stands by diligently, ready to initiate the flow of stress hormones cortisol and adrenalin (also called epinephrine) into your body and mind when it perceives possible danger.

When there has been chronic and/or life-threatening trauma, the amygdala can go into overdrive, perceiving danger when there is none. When this happens, you stay revved up, possibly for years. Your body acts as if it is in a danger zone, when in actuality there is no impending threat in the environment around you. Additionally, when your amygdala remembers that the people closest to you hurt you, it may, quite naturally, unconsciously steer you away from intimate relationships or direct you toward relationships that are equally unnurturing.

Also part of the limbic system, the *hippocampus* sits next to your amygdala. Your hippocampus, which helps you to remember, grasp ideas, and learn skills, is very susceptible to stress. Your hippocampus has many receptors for cortisol (a stress hormone). When your amygdala sends out the message to activate your fight-flight-freeze response, your hippocampus gets flooded with cortisol, which makes comprehension or recall of information difficult.

Ongoing high stress inhibits your ability to study and store information. In fact, according to Victor Carrión (2010) and others, ongoing stress in early life can decrease the size of your hippocampus. However, there is hope. The hippocampus is capable of growing new neurons, and nothing is known to be superior to regular aerobic exercise for activating neuronal growth. (Of course, you have to continually be engaged in novel learning to make use of those new neurons. Otherwise, they are unneeded and cast off. Reading this book and practicing yoga make use of new neurons!) Yoga practices help to preserve your hippocampus by activating your relaxation response, which dramatically reduces the amount of cortisol pumped into your system.

Cortex and Prefrontal Cortex

The third brain region in review is the *cortex*, which is not fully developed, in size or capacity, at birth. During infancy through the toddler years your cortex grew and created many neuronal connections as you learned numerous skills, including how to walk, use the toilet, feed and dress yourself, speak, and communicate with others. This part of your brain was influenced by your childhood home environment and surrounding culture as it took in which language(s) were spoken, how foods were seasoned, and how much laughter and love was expressed.

At the front of your cortex, generally above and behind your eyebrows, is your remarkable prefrontal cortex. The most recently evolved brain region, it does not reach full maturity until you are in your midtwenties. Not only does it have vast neuronal connections with every other part of the brain, its capacity and function responds to the learning environment it is in. It is also greatly influenced by your experiences, including childhood maltreatment (Lanius 2010).

Also called *the area of executive control*, this brain region allows you to be intentional. It helps you make wise decisions rather than making choices based on impulse or habit, such as when you choose to go to bed at a reasonable hour when exhausted instead of staying up late and watching television like you usually do. When you deliberately focus, such as you are doing right now, while reading, your prefrontal cortex reduces distraction by restraining brain regions that take in other sensory input. This prevents your attention from being diverted to other familiar sights, sounds, and smells, such as the sight of a pet walking across the floor. When concentrating, the prefrontal cortex also quiets your mind so that it generates fewer thoughts. (After all, you cannot focus when distracted by thoughts about the future or past.)

However, when frightened, your attention is hijacked by the need for safety. For example, if you hear someone loudly banging on the door, you stop reading and do what is needed to maintain your well-being and possibly the safety of others. Reading a book is optional; tending to your immediate physical survival is not. Also, the racing and scattered thoughts associated with worry and fear make it next to impossible to concentrate because, being highly evocative, they demand attention. When you are emotionally upset, decisions are made based on the immediate need to somehow settle mind and body. Prefrontal activities of making well-thought-out decisions or instituting purposeful changes are sacrificed for real or perceived preoccupation with safety.

The meditation and yoga practices discussed throughout this book profoundly influence your trainable prefrontal lobe, as they help you to concentrate, slow down the rate of thoughts, and feel calm in your body.

Autonomic Nervous System Arousal and Trauma

The autonomic nervous system, briefly introduced earlier under brain stem, has two primary divisions that act in opposition to each other to help your heart, lungs, and digestive tract function well. One division, the *sympathetic nervous system*, accelerates heart rate, raises blood pressure, and prepares your body to fight or flee. The other, the *parasympathetic system*, slows heart rate and activates your relaxation response. Real and perceived threats of danger dramatically affect this system quickly and automatically. You do not have to instruct your body to prepare for danger; it does so automatically via your nervous system.

Basically, when the amygdala interprets danger, the autonomic nervous system has three choices in how it responds. These three responses involve an activated sympathetic nervous system response, which revs up your body to do what it needs to do to stay alive. When there is time to flee, you run for your life. If there is no time to flee but you have strength enough to fight, you defend yourself. With neither time to flee nor strength to fight, your body goes into a freeze response. Also called *tonic immobility*, freeze response is an experience of simultaneous sympathetic and parasympathetic arousal.

When this freeze response occurs, you feel numb and unable to move or scream. You may also feel cold and disconnected from yourself and your immediate surroundings. This is your body's automatic response, not one you consciously select (Gallop 1977; Levine 2010). In this state you experience less pain or fear. Your body is more apt to go into a state of tonic immobility when the trauma is potentially life threatening (Badosi, Toribioz, Garcia-Graui 2008). You could think of it as a compassionate response from a nervous system that either hopes you will not be harmed if you are inert or prepares you for possible death by dulling your senses. Women, not as physically strong as men and typically less able to fight or flee, experience this freeze response more than men (Blanchard et al. 2002).

As you recall, the amygdala's job is to ensure survival. When it is chronically activated by abuse, neglect, violence, or other calamity, it goes into overdrive, misinterpreting nonthreatening stimuli as dangerous. Then, more and more of life, including relationships, feels unsafe. Your body tells you life is not safe and your thoughts agree with your body. In Peter Levine's words (2010, 183), "If our muscles and guts are set to respond to danger, then our mind will tell us that we have something to fear." The body and mind mutually influence and act as one. This, when perpetuated, is how the trauma response lives on long after the danger has passed.

This type of communication between body and mind, when it is ongoing, results in your nervous system staying revved up. Your body becomes less able to relax and you remain tense and frightened. In addition to causing emotional distress and fewer close relationships, sympathetic nervous system dominance leads to major health problems such as heart disease and chronic illnesses. No wonder adversity in early life is closely linked with health problems (Felitti et al. 1998).

This body-mind communication impacts how you live. In the aftermath of damaging relationship trauma, the amygdala and your thoughts may conspire to keep you safe by steering you away from the possibility of future intimacy. Not knowing that they are perpetuating an outdated trauma response that no longer serves well-being, the amygdala and your thoughts keep on attempting to keep you out of harm's way. Although their inner dialogue is understandable, the consequences of a revved-up nervous system and persistent thoughts about how you cannot trust people are painful.

To help you recognize sympathetic and parasympathetic nervous system dominance we lay out what happens in body and mind when each one prevails.

Sympathetic Nervous System Dominance

Nicknamed the *fight-or-flight system*, it allows your body to function under stress. Following is a list of what happens during sympathetic dominance.

- Elevated heart rate

- Chronic muscle tension (body prepared to fight or flee with no release of energy)

- Increased threat perception (life seems more dangerous)

- Diminished neocortical functioning (can't think clearly or focus)

- Loss of language and speech (blood diverted from cortex to fear center)

- Fearful or angry emotions

- Reactivity (emotional reactions vs. reasoned action)

- Perpetuation of anxiety and traumatic stress (mutual reinforcement: body says "I'm afraid," mind says, "there must be something to be afraid of," body says "I'm ready to run or fight")

- High brain-wave activity (thoughts race and are scattered, focusing is difficult)

Parasympathetic Nervous System Dominance

Nicknamed the *rest-and-digest system*, it helps your body to return to a balanced state after experiencing stress. Following is a list of what happens during parasympathetic dominance.

- Optimal or normal heart rate

- Muscles relax (body feels comfortable)

- Decreased threat perception (life seems safer)

- Peak cognitive performance (can learn, reason, make wise decisions)

- Ability to speak about and make sense of experiences (optimal blood flow to cortex)

- Ability to regulate and handle a range of emotions

- Intentionality (reasoned actions vs. emotional reactivity)

- Positive social engagement (desire to seek pleasant and intimate contact)

- Ability to cultivate sense of inner calm, reset nervous system to optimal functioning

- Low brain-wave activity (thoughts focus, mental clarity)

Autonomic Nervous System Dysregulation

This is so important that we repeat it again. The trauma response is not the result of conscious choice. It is truly physical, based on the response of the autonomic nervous system. Therefore, it makes sense that persistent hyperarousal of the sympathetic nervous system is one of the diagnostic criteria of a PTSD and the most characteristic sign of arousal in PTSD is elevated heart rate (Martinez et al. 2010). If the trauma response is not worked out of the nervous system, it becomes dysregulated, stuck in a chronic pattern of being amped up, whereby you feel afraid and ready to fight or flee, or stuck in an immobilization response, whereby you feel exhausted, numb, and disinterested in life.

Autonomic Nervous System Regulation with Yoga

Healing from trauma involves helping your body to let go of these seemingly fixed patterns. Your nervous system needs to be reset so that your sympathetic and parasympathetic nervous systems work together optimally, allowing you to fully rest at night, be comfortably alert during the day, and feel highly energized when needed. Doing a simple yoga practice more days than not, one that includes comfortable stretches, focused breathing, and a few minutes of meditation, can help to normalize your heart rate and reset your autonomic nervous system.

Research helps verify the benefits of yoga. Dhanunjaya Lakkireddy (2011) found yoga to be an effective treatment for individuals with irregular heart rates (atrial fibrillation). Participants in the study who practiced yoga also reported decreased anxiety and depression. Since there is a significant relationship between maltreatment in early life, heart disease, and emotional distress, this study, while not specifically about trauma, speaks to the healing value of yoga for people with histories of trauma. Plus, as you are about to read, yoga's profound effect on heart rate reduces the lingering effects that trauma has on the autonomic nervous system.

Heart-Rate Variability

Your heart has been beating since you were in your mother's womb and will continue to do so until you die. How healthily it beats (and perhaps how long you live) is utterly dependent upon the synergistic relationship of the sympathetic and parasympathetic branches of your autonomic nervous systems. Like a throttle, your sympathetic branch increases your heart's action and, like a brake, your parasympathetic branch slows it down. The interplay between the two produces an ongoing increase and decrease in heart rate. Your heart is designed to beat at an ever-changing, not fixed, rate so that it can respond to the commands of your nervous system. One way to determine what is happening in your autonomic nervous system is to measure your heart-rate variability (HRV), which is derived from an electrocardiogram. HRV, which represents the changes in the distance between one heartbeat and the next, is measured by the variation in the beat-to-beat interval. The spaces between heartbeats are not identical.

Decreased activity in the parasympathetic branch contributes to increased activity in the sympathetic branch, which results in reduced HRV. Low HRV has significant relationship to PTSD. This is not surprising, considering that the nervous system remains in high gear, ready to fight or flee, long after the actual threat is gone. Your heart ends up working overtime and ineffectively.

Optimal Heart-Rate Variability

Optimal HRV usually occurs when you are in a relaxed mental state, emotionally calm, and breathing fully and comfortably, in the five- to seven-breaths-per-minute range. Yoga, with its emphasis on steady, easy breathing, increases activity in the parasympathetic nervous system and increases HRV. In fact, in its Mental Health Letter of April 2009, Harvard University approved of yoga as a treatment for anxiety and PTSD due to the increase of HRV resulting from practicing yoga. That same year, Terri Zucker (2009) reported a study that found that paced breathing (breathing in for five counts and breathing out for five counts), or about six breaths per minute, was more helpful than progressive muscle relaxation in increasing HRV.

This is encouraging and empowering news. You can intervene on your own behalf, literally alter your HRV, and reverse the effect that trauma has on your nervous system. Try it for yourself. Stop reading for one minute. Literally, pause. Close your eyes and take six breaths, counting to five on your inhalation and five on your exhalation. Notice if your breath deepened and your mind got quiet.

Vagus Nerve

The primary parasympathetic nerve is the *vagus nerve*, also called *cranial nerve* X. Nicknamed the *wandering nerve*, it is the longest nerve in your body, originating at the brain stem and going down through the organs, finally inserting at your pelvis floor. This interesting nerve, operating independently of the spinal cord, is not part of your central nervous system. Eighty percent of its nerve fibers send messages about the state of internal organs, including the heart, to your brain. Not only does it relay information to your brain, it facilitates the functioning of organs, including your heart. In the previous section we discussed how the parasympathetic nerve innervates the heart. This is done by the vagus nerve. Simply stated, your vagus nerve lowers your heart rate.

This remarkable nerve supplies nerve fibers to your throat, voice box, and windpipe. This is why your voice has soothing resonance when you are relaxed and is tight and sometimes shrill when you are frightened. Steven Porges (2011) theorizes that the vagus nerve is an important aspect of your ability to socially engage with others. Porges coined the term *neuroception* to describe the ability of nerve circuits to distinguish whether other people are safe or dangerous. Amazingly, specific areas of the brain detect body and facial movements along with tone of voice to determine whether the person it is assessing is trustworthy. All this occurs autonomically, beneath conscious awareness. This is why, as adults, most people automatically gravitate toward people who feel safe, much in the same way that children run to trusted adults when they are frightened.

Porges suggests that trauma can compromise your ability to recognize safety in someone else. The defensive behaviors triggered by the fight-flight-freeze response remain "on line" and your social engagement system goes "off line." When this happens you feel unsupported, alone, and have difficulty relying on others.

Vagus Nerve and Music Therapy

Steven Porges also recommends music therapy as a way to stimulate this social system. Singing is an experience of vocal expression, whereby intonation and tonal quality reflect the emotional quality of the melody. You can hum soothing sounds, chant comforting words, and sing sweet tunes to reinstate your ability to approach and be soothed by safe relationships. Additionally, when you sing or chant you produce sound during long exhalations, which deepens your breath, countering the rapid breath associated with the fight-or-flight response.

Chanting and singing spiritual songs infuse your body and mind with sacred sounds and vibrations. It also activates your nervous system's relaxation response and your ability to discern safety, thus enabling you to turn to others for support. Singing and chanting in a group has the additional benefit of feeling connected with others while feeling relaxed.

One woman, whose primary yoga practice is devotional prayer, chants the words "Blessed heart of Mary" repeatedly, explaining that those four words draw her deeply inward, past the place of trauma and grief. She said, "Singing this prayer is a great blessing for me because it gives me glimpses of my own loving heart. I repeat the prayer again and again. It reconnects me to my inner goodness and helps me to not feel so bad about myself. It also helps me out of my introversion, enabling me to come out of my bedroom and interact with my husband and daughter."

SINGING, CHANTING, OR HUMMING PRACTICE

Experiment and decide, based on personal appeal, whether you want to sing, chant, or hum. Then select a phrase, song, or melody that warms, uplifts, or soothes you. Consider a short refrain of a spiritual song (perhaps even one you sang as a child), an inspirational saying, a prayer, or a scripture that deeply touches and pleases. Alternatively, select a short melody that stirs your heart and is easy to hum. Keep your song, phrase, or tune brief and easy to repeat. Decide on a time, possibly first thing in the morning, when you can devote a few minutes to this lovely practice. Of course, the benefit comes from a regular practice.

Try this Sanskrit chant: "**Shanti, shanti, shanti, Om.**" Or its English version: "Peace, peace, peace, Om." Alternatively, you can chant "Peace, peace, peace, Amen." To chant, select one musical note. Sing and repeat the chant using one note.

Breath and Your Nervous System

Breath, governed primarily by the autonomic nervous system, is with you every minute of your entire life. Ever reliable, breath takes in new air and expels old air, supplying you with a mixture of oxygen and carbon dioxide. Without your saying "Breathe in, breathe out," breath sustains your life, like a dear friend. Breath is also attuned to your nervous system's commands to fight-flight-freeze or relax. Breath responds to the fight-flight-freeze command by becoming faster and shallower. It remains in high gear as long as needed. Breath responds to the relaxation command by slowing down and becoming deeper to the point that your belly rises on the inhalation and falls on the exhalation.

Breath is also governed by the voluntary nervous system, meaning that you can intentionally alter breath. Once again, breathe in and count to five. Then breathe out and count to five. Notice that your breath becomes unhurried. Doing this releases muscle tension, slows heart rate, increases HRV, and cultivates a sense of inner calm. Learn how to take care of your breath and you help your autonomic nervous system function optimally.

Breath and the Thinking Mind

Pace of breath and speed of thoughts match one another. The brain and body are so interconnected that racing thoughts cause stress hormones (adrenaline and cortisol) to be released, which in turn triggers fast, shallow breath. In the same manner, intentional slow breathing causes the rapid firing of thoughts to subside. You cannot have racing thoughts when you breathe deeply. Breathe deeply and your brain takes additional action by releasing a calming neurotransmitter, called GABA, that further induces relaxation and focus. In fact, Chris Streeter and colleagues (2010) reported on a study comparing yoga and walking as effective ways to reduce anxiety. The researchers found that yoga, with its focus on breathing, had the greater benefit, due to the increased GABA levels measured in the yoga practitioners. As a result, the minds of those practicing yoga became quieter than the minds of the walkers.

Breath and Your Personal Yoga Practice

Pranayama is a Sanskrit word that means "to extend breath or the life force." The yogis of ancient India knew that working with breath is a powerful way to bring health and harmony to the body and mind. They verified the power of *pranayama* through their own experience and touted its benefits long before science explained them. Breathing practices are fundamental to yoga, even more so than the physical poses. *Pranayama*, the heart of yoga, a complete practice in itself, is so central that doing yoga poses without focusing on breath is merely a form of exercise, not the practice of yoga.

You do not have to be physically fit to practice yoga. You do not need to attend a class to begin yoga. Start with a very simple breathing practice in your home. Select a quiet, comfortable place, perhaps a favorite chair by a window or fireplace. If you are ill or physically disabled, you can certainly do this in bed. Prop up with pillows as desired for comfort.

Dedicate a few minutes to taking care of your breath. Early morning is wonderful, as it sets the tone for the day, but any consistent time that fits into your daily schedule is great. Pick a time and place that works well, and do the practice in a way that is as comforting as putting on a sweater when you are chilled.

MEASURED BREATHING PRACTICE

Sit or recline. Feel your feet on the floor and your hips on the chair, or feel the sensations of your body lying in your bed. To prepare for measured breathing, take a nice breath in and gently blow it out through pursed lips. Then, counting with your fingers, breathe in for five counts and breathe out for five counts. Repeat for five or ten times. Stay in your comfort zone. There is no benefit in breathing in a way that distresses you.

You may stop here. Your commitment and willingness to take care of your breath is what is most important. Add on to your practice gradually in the same way you step up your walking distance to increase your level of physical fitness.

GENTLE BREATH-RETENTION PRACTICE

When you are ready, you may add a gentle breath-retention practice. Before beginning, we again stress the importance of staying in your comfort zone. Start easy. Breathe in for four counts, hold your breath for four counts, and breathe out for eight counts. After a couple of cycles, lengthen your breath retention. Breathe in for four counts, hold your breath for seven counts, and breathe out for eight counts. Do this a few times. There is no hurry. Give yourself some time to become acclimated to this breathing. It is truly tranquilizing medicine for your nervous system.

Breathe to Regulate Your Emotions

Physiologically, you cannot be highly anxious or angry when you intentionally breathe deeply. However, the energy of anxiety and anger is intense, like an undertow in the water that sweeps you away from shore. When you are overwrought you may not remember to breath deeply if you do not have an established breathing practice. If you follow through with a daily practice of even a few minutes, you not only recondition your breath but help train your body to remember to breathe through distress.

You do not have to be at the mercy of runaway anxiety or irritability. You do not have to suffer relentlessly. Intervene and help yourself. Practice measured breathing regularly so that when you are upset you can breathe in for a count of five and breathe out for a count of five at least five times.

Summary

If you are like most, when you think of trauma, you think of life-threatening, horrific events. However, the most prevalent form of trauma is emotional maltreatment between family members.

Damaging to everyone involved, the effects can last for a lifetime. Trauma leaves imprints on body and mind that, left untreated, can result in poor health and unhappiness.

We have learned from science how trauma can affect your brain and nervous system. Fundamentally, trauma leaves your nervous system in a trauma-ready state, not just for a while but as a way of functioning and being. Research is now verifying that working with your breath to deepen your inhalation and lengthen your exhalation engages your relaxation response, quiets your worried mind, and gently releases the embedded trauma response from your body and brain.

chapter 4

healing trauma with a physical practice of yoga

therapeutic yoga is enjoyable and easy to do for most people. You do not have to be athletic, flexible, or experienced in yoga. Plus, if you have physical limitations, simply do the poses that are appropriate for you. It is healing to spend a little time doing poses, and we encourage you to do what you can. All you need before you begin is a yoga mat, a couple of small folded blankets, and the instructions outlined in this chapter.

We approach this chapter systematically so that you appreciate how healing the physical practice of yoga is. Taking it step-by-step, we first describe muscular tension. Next we describe how emotions are held in the body. After that we orient you to emotional-spiritual energy centers, called *chakras* in yoga philosophy, and look at how trauma impacts chakras. Last, we present a series of poses and a way of practicing them that works emotional trauma out of your body. Before going into this material, though, we want to offer a little perspective.

Yoga is a profound ritual of self-care. And, of course, you already do some forms of self-care. You bathe, brush your teeth, and tend to the surface of your body. Taking care of your body inside of your skin is just as essential, which is what yoga does. The physical practice of yoga takes care of your bones, muscles, emotions, and a whole lot more.

For the record, we want to say that performing self-care is not something you earn the right to do. You need not justify self-care or think that you have to do good acts to be worthy of it. You do self-care because of how it affects you. You respond to self-care the way water lilies respond to water and sunny skies. They bloom, not because they deserve to, but because it is their nature to. So, when you practice physical yoga, you do far more than just stretch your muscles. You transform body and emotions into an environment that promotes healing and well-being.

Your nervous system learns how to relax and muscles become stronger and suppler. However, when carefully designed, your practice also gently releases old emotional pain because, as distinct as they may feel, emotions are utterly intertwined with your physical body. A product of the interaction between body, mind, and spirit, they are physiological expressions that you experience in your muscles and energy. The following examples are overly simplified, because there can be much variation; however, they demonstrate how emotions show up in your body. Muscles generally feel weak when you are afraid, tense when you are angry, and heavy when you are depressed. You also experience emotions energetically. Fear causes your body's energy to tremble, anger makes it clench, and depression causes it to stagnate. Since yoga postures work with your body, a faithful practice of yoga cleanses your body from long-held painful emotional patterns, allowing you to feel increasingly at home in your body and relaxed.

Finally, a compassionate physical practice makes you conscious of your spiritual nature. You already and always are a spiritual being, but when your body and mind are upset it is easy to overlook. As powerful as spiritual presence is, it can feel subtle in comparison to obvious physical and emotional pain. If your body has been mistreated and degraded, it may feel uncomfortable and unwelcoming. Going to your yoga mat, regardless of your size or shape, sends a message deep inside that you matter. Returning to your mat day after day becomes a place where you tend to your body and spirit.

Muscular Tension and Yoga

You have approximately 640 skeletal muscles in your body. They support your joints, hold your body upright, and move your bones. Without them you would be utterly immobile. Their tasks are complex, yet their actions are simple. Muscles have one action. They contract, or shorten, when they receive the message from your central nervous system to do so. When the signal ceases, muscles effortlessly lengthen, returning to a resting state, unless they have forgotten how to relax.

Muscle tension, created when muscles continuously pull, is the outcome of chronically held stress. A tight muscle is a muscle contraction that does not release fully after it stops receiving the message to work from your brain. The muscle remains partially contracted and does not allow muscle tone to drop to zero in a resting state. When this happens you are not able to voluntarily relax your muscle. According to Thomas Hanna (1988), muscle tone may remain anywhere from 10 percent, causing the muscle to feel tired and firm, to 40 percent, whereby the muscle feels hard and painful.

A yoga practice releases muscular tension. Standing poses require muscular effort, which burns up stored tension and enables muscles to relax. Seated poses gently stretch muscles, showing them how to let go. Longer-held restorative poses, whereby you lie on the floor, perhaps supported by a folded blanket or bolster, feel safe and allow your body to relax.

Emotions and Your Physical Body

Emotions, when you are able to experience them moving through you, let you feel fully human. You are probably more familiar with some emotions than others. Often this is the case, especially in the aftermath of trauma when fear, anger, confusion, and sadness are intense and/or long lasting. When one or two emotions are strong you may be less able to experience a full range of emotions, especially ones that are subtle and sweet. Healing involves learning to let emotions move on through and experiencing many emotions, including delight. We want for you to be able to give a personalized expression of joy, such as this one, given by a friend: "It's like my mind and body are humming together, taking in the perfection of the moment."

The more you understand about emotions, the easier it is to let them be without getting stuck in them. Emotions express the intimacy of body, mind, and spirit. Sometimes we say that body and mind join together in holy wedlock and create emotions. As such, emotions are a natural part of human life. They are neither weakness nor flaw and are designed to be experienced and let be, not denied, made wrong, or ignored. Emotions originate from different physiological/mental states. Fear and anger, the survival emotions, arise when perceived or real needs for safety, approval, and control seem threatened. Other emotional states, such as peace and bliss, arise from feeling connected to stillness and other spiritual energies such as oneness and pure love.

When the bodily sensations associated with emotions are unbearable, it is adaptive to push them into unconsciousness, so that you do not notice that which is more than you can cope with. You forget or become unaware. This is what vulnerable children or, more accurately, their nervous systems, naturally tend to do when exposed to maltreatment. Adults exposed to trauma often have the same nervous system response. This dissociative, or tuning-out, response, although temporarily helpful, garbles communication between body and mind. Emotions and physical sensations go underground. However, they live on and they work on you. Your body and mind still communicate, even if you cannot decode their messages. Dreams, snatches of memory, and traces of sensations break through, letting you know emotions are there.

Emotions as Motivators

Emotions, whether you are conscious of them or they are buried in your unconscious, motivate behaviors. Fear seeks safety, sadness seeks relief, anger seeks revenge, and joy seeks expression. When emotions such as fear go underground, they can show up as enduring characteristics of your personality without your knowing why.

Unconsciously, they motivate behaviors and fuel self-perpetuating traits until they are acknowledged.

Here is an example of one way that fear showed up in Mary's personality. Mary subconsciously believed that she was unworthy of love. Therefore she feared that she would be abandoned by those she loved. Fear motivated her to be nonassertive in her intimate relationships. Since fear seeks safety, relationship security was of top importance to her. As a result she dismissed her emotions and needs and focused on pleasing others. "Preparing to express conflict still causes my heart to race," Mary explains. "However, I know that nonassertiveness builds resentment, which sucks the life out of intimacy and reinforces my old narrative of unworthiness. So, after mulling it over and breathing deeply to steady my trembling, I cough up the words that express what I need to say."

Energy Centers

Clearly, there is more to you than thoughts, emotions, and your physical body. You are also energy. You have already read about how emotional and mental tension is interwoven into muscular tension. Psychological and spiritual energy also live in your physical body and, while energy in your body cannot be seen, it can be measured. For example, a sensitive instrument measures the electromagnetic field that radiates within and beyond the body from the heart. According to Doc Childre and Howard Martin (1999), the Institute of HeartMath has found that your heart is responsive to emotional energies. Emotions change the way your heart beats. Anger and frustration are linked with erratic heart rhythms, and love is connected with coherent heart rhythms. These changes in heart rate show up in the electromagnetic field. Your heart communicates information about your emotions up to your brain and throughout your body through a variety of ways, including its electromagnetic field.

Long before technology gave scientists the ability to measure energy, the ancient yogis perceived the energetic basis of matter. They charted the movement of energy in the human body and outlined seven centers called *chakras*, or force centers, of psycho-spiritual energies that form around the main nerve plexus of the spine. In Alan Finger's words (2005, 17), "the chakras are where we receive, assimilate, and distribute our life energies. Through external situations or internal habits a chakra can become unbalanced." Imagine seven whirlpools of psychological matter and great spiritual potential swirling around in front of your spine gathering up and dispersing your life energy.

These natural energy vortexes are impacted by life experiences. In the same way that your body shivers when a cold wind blows, you respond emotionally and spiritually to what happens to you. When this energy gets trapped inside, then, unbeknownst to you, old emotional and mental tensions intercept and direct your life energy. Obviously, these tensions include the undeniable imprints of trauma. Fortunately, you are not doomed to a life that is patterned by old, unprocessed emotional energy.

A well-designed yoga practice releases trapped psychological energy and connects you to spiritual energies such as forgiveness, understanding, and profound acceptance. Before showing you a series of yoga poses that help balance your emotional-spiritual energy centers, we want to give you a little information about each of the chakras. That way you can make a direct connection between the poses and healing residual trauma.

Seven Chakras

Following is a listing of each of the chakras along with their basic physical, mental, emotional, and spiritual concerns. This is a brief overview, containing just enough information to help you appreciate the relationship between trauma and the chakra energies without going into a lot of detail. If you would like more thorough explorations of the chakras, we recommend the writings of Swami Ajaya (1983), Anodea Judith (1996), and Alan Finger (2005).

To begin, imagine each chakra as a wheel of energy. Each of the seven spinning wheels is a field of energy that contains certain physical, mental, emotional, and spiritual content. The first chakra sits at the base of your spine and the seventh chakra is at the top, or crown, of your head. The other chakras are arranged vertically along the spine, in between the first and seventh chakras.

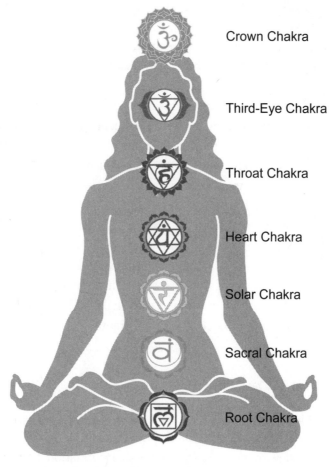

Crown Chakra

Third-Eye Chakra

Throat Chakra

Heart Chakra

Solar Chakra

Sacral Chakra

Root Chakra

Image copyright © Surabhi25/Shutterstock.com, 2012. Used under license from Shutterstock.com.

The lower three energy centers pertain to basic human survival. They are responsible for your self-image and how you relate to the world around you. The upper three energy centers pertain to your mind and spirituality. Right in the middle, in the area of your heart, the fourth energy center is where energies of higher consciousness, including compassion and insight, tend to the wounds of your lifetime, lifting them from darkness into the light of understanding.

- **The root chakra**, also called the base chakra, is the first energy center. It's located at the base of your spine. Its basic concerns are survival and stability. This pertains to your needs for safety and security, not only physical but emotional as well. Maltreatment and neglect in early life and life-threatening traumas at any age obviously disrupt your ability to trust that life is safe enough and/or that you have the capacity to protect yourself. If you experience a lot of fear, you may have imbalance in this center. Things done for self-preservation—such as recoiling from involvement in life, seeking security above all else, binge eating, stubborn tendencies, and hoarding—may result from life energy being processed through fear.

- **The sacral chakra** is the second energy center, located at the lower abdomen, between belly button and pubic bone. Its basic concerns are sexuality, creativity, and relationships. Sexual abuse interferes with the vitality and ingenuity that make life interesting. If you are prone to guilt, feel inhibited or numb, or feel emotionally and sexually out of control, you may have imbalances in this center. Behaviors engaged in for self-gratification, such as addictions and emotional dependency on others, may result from life energy being processed through guilt.

- **The solar chakra** is located at the solar plexus, between belly button and bottom of rib cage. This is the third energy center. Its basic concerns are personal power, self-esteem, willfulness, and energy. Emotional maltreatment that dishonors or degrades leaves the stain of shame that taints self-worth. If you are predisposed toward feeling powerless, have issues with control, or suffer from low self-esteem, you may have imbalances in this center. Behaviors that reflect uncertainty about personal power—such as poor follow-through, passivity, or the need to be right or domineering—may result from life energy being processed through underlying feelings of shame.

- **The heart chakra** is the fourth center. Located at the heart center, its basic concerns are love, compassion, acceptance, and trust. Overwhelming rejection, betrayal, and loss take a toll on the human heart and intimate relationships. If you are prone toward isolation, emotional coldness, emotional dependency, or emotional reactivity, you may have imbalances in this center. Behaviors that indicate closed-heartedness, difficulty with forgiveness, and fear of abandonment or of being loved may result from life energy being processed through underlying feelings of grief.

- **The throat chakra**, the fifth center, is located at the throat. Its basic concerns are communication, inspiration, expression, and faith. Being yelled at, lied to, and overly criticized disrupts the capacity to recognize truth and to speak forthrightly. If you tend to be shy, fear speaking assertively, interrupt others in conversation, or talk without saying much you may have imbalances in this center. Communication that distorts, hints, hides, and overrides may result from life energy being processed through a squelching of the basic impulse to self-express.

- **The third-eye chakra** is located between the eyebrows, just above the bridge of the nose. The sixth center, its basic concerns are psychic, emotional, and mental intelligence and intuition. Chaotic, uncertain, or dangerous environments that leave you believing that you cannot trust what you see or that teach you that what you see is not true disturb your capacity to discern the real from the unreal. If you find it difficult to imagine the future or remember the past, or suffer from nightmares or obsessions, you may have imbalances in this center. Delusions of persecution, dogmatic beliefs, difficulty accessing intuition, and having little imagination may result from life energy being processed through false views about what is real.

- **The crown chakra** is the seventh center, located at the top of the head. Its basic concerns are devotion, inspiration, selflessness, and spiritual understanding. Forced religiosity, beliefs that the physical body or emotions are bad, and obedience that forbids questioning thwart the felt sense of connection with higher consciousness. If you are highly cynical, adhere to rigid beliefs, tend to intellectualize or feel disconnected from your body, you may have imbalances in this center. Certainty about who or what God is, excessive materialism, disdain toward the spiritual, and aversion to other faiths may result from life energy being processed through blinding attachment to religious ideas.

To optimize the benefits of your practice, we are going to present a sequence of yoga poses for trauma, taking the chakra perspective into consideration. We begin with poses for chakra one and end with poses for chakra seven. This way, while doing the poses, you can appreciate and be aware of balancing your psycho-spiritual physical energies. We recommend a comprehensive yoga practice that addresses all the chakras, because, if you are like most people, you probably identified, at least to some degree, with all of the concerns described in this section. However, you may want to adapt your practice to focus primarily on one or two chakra areas that you sense need extra attention.

Important Considerations for Your Yoga Practice

Nonviolence is central to yoga. Most important, do no harm and do not force your body. Yoga is a practice that unites body, mind, and breath. Respect all three so that you feel comfortable in them and they feel safe with you. Listen to your body and energy. When you are tired, go easy on standing poses and stay longer in floor poses. On other days, when you have more energy, remain in the standing poses long enough to feel heat. This is purifying, as it burns up stored tension. Afterward, give yourself sufficient time in seated or supine poses to reset your nervous system. This allows you to fully relax and remind your body that ease is a natural state of being.

Adapt the practice to suit your needs. If you are in the aftermath of recent trauma, be especially sensitive to your energy. Go to your mat as an act of carving out time to take care of yourself. (Remember: You need tender care in the same way a lily needs the sun. If you have been hurt by another, deep inside you may yearn for someone else to take care of you and not want to do it for yourself.) Some days you may only feel up to doing two or three seated or lying-down poses and then feel ready for rest. Conclude your practice by covering yourself with a blanket and resting with your eyes closed. Do poses that promote feelings of safety and being supported. Give yourself some recovery time. Then, when you are ready, try some standing poses to determine if you are ready to build stamina. It is very empowering to develop muscular strength if you feel beaten down by past trauma. You might also benefit from a vigorous practice that builds resolve. If your heart feels broken, begin gently and gradually increase the time you spend in the heart-opening poses.

Adapting the Practice for Your Emotional Response to Trauma

Some people, especially women, are prone to dissociation in response to trauma. If this describes you, you may be attracted to a flowing, moving practice yet really benefit from dedicating a significant portion of your practice to seated and floor poses that allow you to become still. Some people are prone to depression in response to trauma. If you relate to this, you may prefer a gentle, slow-moving practice yet respond well to an energizing, strong practice that moves sluggish energy through the body. Others are prone to anger in response to trauma. If you identify with this, you might like your practice to be strong and muscular, yet benefit from including cooling, restorative poses.

Adapting the Practice for Your Body-Mind Type

It is also helpful to consider your body-mind type in doing yoga poses. If you are slender, quick moving, and fast thinking, you may be attracted to moving rapidly through your yoga poses. Yet it may be more balancing to stay in poses for a while and focus on breathing, to allow your body to slow down and your mind to quiet. If you are a muscular and determined type, you may gravitate toward poses that build muscle and show mastery, yet may profit from flowing from one pose to the next, in rhythm with soft music, so that you feel your gentler side. If you are prone to carrying extra weight and are a slow, methodical type of person, you might find seated and resting poses desirable, yet may respond really well to focusing more on standing poses that increase strength and energy.

You will return to your practice again and again if you enjoy it. Therefore, do accommodate your preferences. Begin your session in the manner that you inevitably gravitate toward, but do experiment with the body-mind-type considerations we laid out. The idea is to balance your energy centers rather than reinforcing old tendencies that can aggravate your overall sense of well-being or inhibit recovery.

Preparing for Yoga

Dress in comfortable, stretchy clothes. Select a calm, pleasant room or outdoor space where you will be undisturbed. Lay out a yoga mat and have one or two folded blankets nearby, along with an upholstered pillow or bolster if you like. Keep this book nearby so you can follow along while you are learning the series.

Before beginning, promise yourself that you will listen to your body so that you practice in a way that is pleasing to you. The biggest clue about the benefit and appropriateness of any particular pose is your breath. Breathing comfortably is fundamental, so practice in a way that promotes deep, even breathing. If you experience exhaustion or sharp pain, stop and rest. If you have injuries or physical limitations, consult with your physician before attempting these poses.

Incorporate Mantras into Your Practice

We include a mantra, or sacred utterance, that you repeat for each of the seven chakras in the series of poses that follow. Each mantra affirms a simple yet profound truth that, when recited, puts your mind at ease, soothes your emotions, and orients you to the transcendent.

A PRACTICE OF YOGA POSES

Begin your yoga practice with one or both of the following two poses, which are designed to center and calm you. Then begin mindful breathing. Starting with these poses prepares your body and mind for the healing that occurs when you do the rest of your yoga practice.

Comforting Seated Pose

Begin your practice by connecting to yourself and your breath. Sit upright on your yoga mat or a blanket with your legs crossed comfortably in front of you. Place one hand on your heart area and one hand just above your navel. Notice the warmth of your hand on your chest and on your belly. Begin to be aware of your breath. Sit quietly and focus on taking five easy breaths.

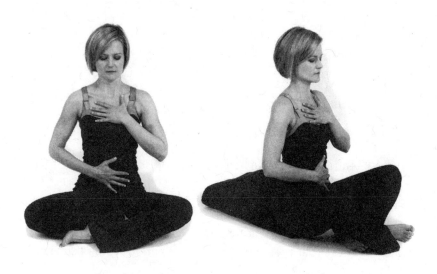

Child's Pose

Get on your hands and knees, with your knees wider than your hips and your feet close together. Then rest your hips on your heels in the pose of a child. Rest your chest on a folded blanket, if you like. Position your arms comfortably in front of you. Place your head gently to one side. Notice where your body touches the floor. Let yourself relax. The floor will support you. Begin to be aware of your breath. Rest quietly and focus on taking five easy breaths.

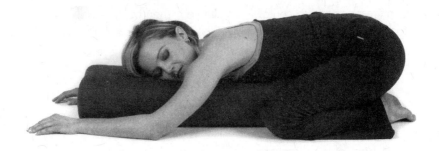

Chakra 1

- **Purpose:** To feel safe and solid, knowing that your feet are under you.

- **Mantra:** "I am safe."

- Begin by reading or chanting **"I am safe."**

- **Intention:** Go through this series of standing poses to develop physical strength.

Choose if you want to practice some or all of these standing poses. Focus on breathing in and out through your nose as you stand in each of the poses. Let your breath be comfortable and full yet not strained.

Crescent Lunge Pose

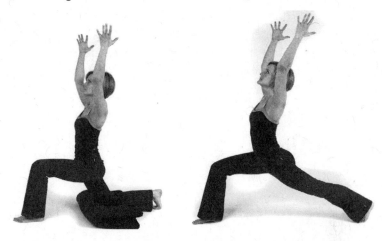

Modified Crescent Lunge Pose

Begin with crescent lunge or modified crescent lunge as pictured. For safety, check that your front knee is right above your front foot, not in front of or behind it. Your back leg may be straight or it may be resting flat on the floor starting at the knee. Arms are raised, but keep shoulders relaxed and down. Focus on breathing in and out as you stand in the pose.

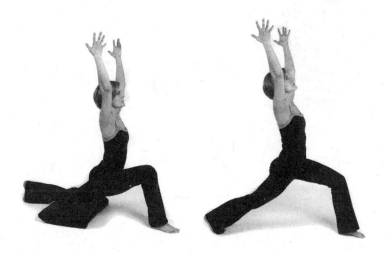

In chair pose, you can have your knees and feet close together or about hip-width apart. From a standing position, lower yourself gently as if sitting into a chair. Raise your arms above your head, but keep your shoulders down. Watch to ensure that your knees are directly above your feet, not in front of them. Avoiding leaning your torso forward.

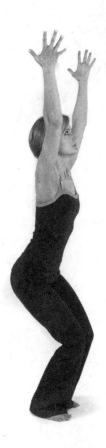

Goddess Pose

To go into goddess pose, stand facing the long side of your mat. Place your feet one leg-length apart from each other, or a little closer for comfort. Angle your feet so they point toward the front corners of your mat. Keeping your back straight and upright, bend your knees, looking to see that they are directly over your feet, not in front of them. Position your arms out at your sides at shoulder height. Bend your elbows into "cactus arms" and point your fingers toward the sky. Take five to ten comfortable breaths. If this position hurts your knees, straighten your legs. If this position hurts your arms or shoulders, drop your arms to your sides or raise your arms overhead. Breathe.

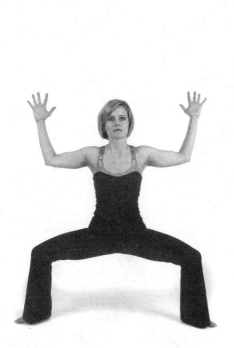
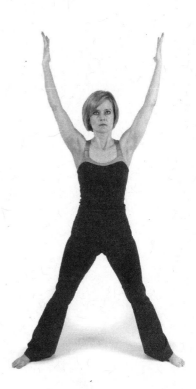

Side Warrior Pose

To go into side warrior pose, stand facing the long side of your mat. Place your feet one leg-length apart. Point your right foot toward the top of the mat and your left foot at a forty-five degree angle toward your right foot, as you see modeled in the picture. Without forcing, face your hips squarely toward the long side of the mat. Bend your right knee, checking to make sure that it is positioned directly above your ankle. Extend your arms out at shoulder height. Lower your shoulders a little bit and let them relax. Look softly over your right hand. Take five to ten comfortable breaths and switch to your left side. To make the pose less strenuous and to protect your bended knee, position your feet a little closer together and bend your knee less.

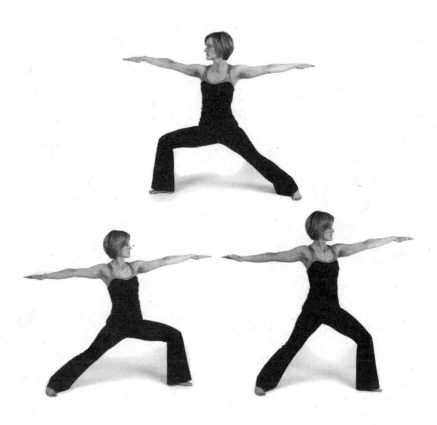

Chakra 2

- **Purpose:** To let yourself move, experience vitality, and enjoy being in your body.

- **Mantra:** "I am alive."

- Begin by reading or chanting **"I am alive."**

- **Intention:** Slowly flow through these poses in an enjoyable way.

Select one or more of the following flowing movements for your practice. Let yourself take pleasure in doing these next poses.

Goddess Pose Flow

You have already done goddess pose, now synchronize the illustrated arm movements with bending and straightening your knees as demonstrated in the photo. Start from standing then, on an exhalation, slowly bend your knees and arms. Raise back to standing on an inhalation. Repeat five or more times, flowing your movement with your breath.

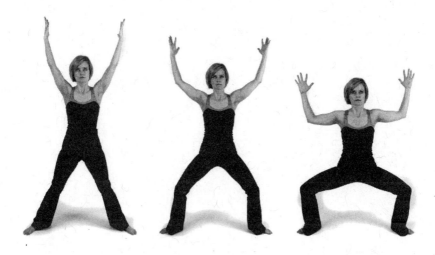

Standing Hip Circles

Stand with your feet hip-width apart or a little more, depending on your comfort. Place your hands on your hips and enjoy making clockwise circles with your hips for a minute or so. Play with creating large and small circles and vary your speed. Then switch direction.

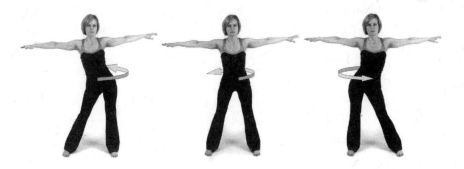

Forward Fold

Select the forward fold that is most comfortable for you. Depending on your body size, you may like your feet fairly close together or spaced hip-width or more apart. You might prefer your knees slightly bent if you are less flexible or have lower-back discomfort. You might prefer legs straight if you are very flexible. Place your arms in the position that feels best to you. Clasping your hands behind your back is more challenging. If you choose this arm position, first interlock your fingers behind your back, then raise your arms, with elbows bent or straight, as far as feels comfortable. Stay in this pose for five or more breaths.

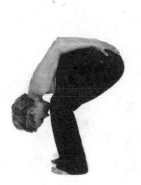
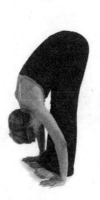
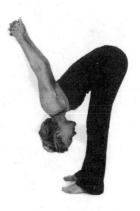

Forward Fold Flow

Once you have found which forward fold pose resonates with you, try a flowing sequence, going back and forth from standing up to bending over. Start from standing, with arms raised above your head. Then on an exhale, bend your knees and fold from your hips. Allow your arms to float down and ultimately rest in whatever position most suits you. On an inhale, slowly unfold back to standing. Do three to six repetitions, as long as it feels enjoyable.

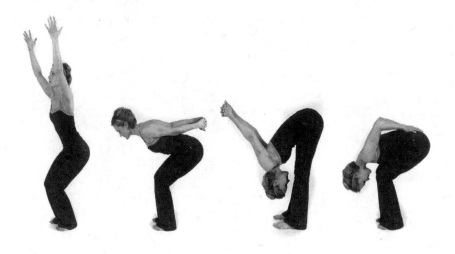

Forward Fold Flow End

Conclude the forward fold flow series with a comfortable forward fold. Stay in it and breathe for five or more breaths. Experiment with letting your exhalations be longer than your inhalations.

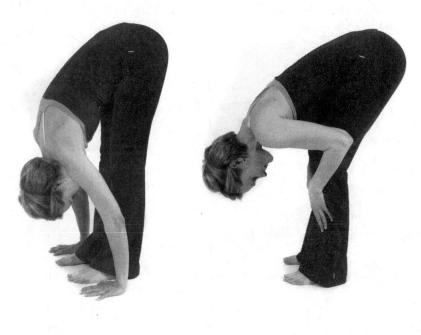

Chakra 3

- **Purpose:** To let yourself make choices, build resolve, and develop personal power.

- **Mantra:** "I choose."

- Begin by reading or chanting **"I choose."**

- **Intention:** Choose which of the following poses to do and how long to hold them.

Half-Locust Pose

Lie on your tummy. Place arms at your side. For half-locust pose, keep your arms, torso, and chin flat on the floor. On an inhale, raise one leg. Determine how long to hold the pose. See if you can hold for at least five breaths. If you cannot, that is okay—do what is appropriate for you. Lower the leg on an exhale and repeat on the other side.

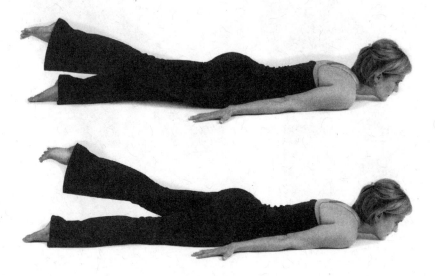

Full-Locust Post

Start in half-locust pose. On an inhale, raise both legs **and** your head and torso. Keep your eyes facing the floor. You may keep your arms down or outstretch them as an extension of your torso. Determine how long to hold the pose. See if you can hold for at least five breaths. If you cannot, that is okay—do what is appropriate for you.

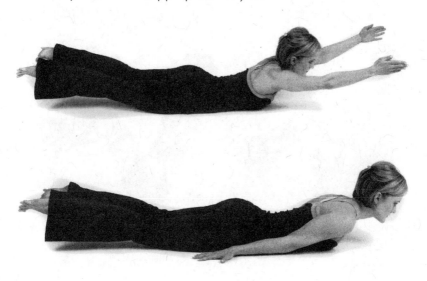

Half-Boat Pose

Sit up with your knees in the air and your feet on the mat to prepare for half-boat pose. Then lift your feet so that you're balancing on your bottom. Place your arms as shown in whichever one of the two poses pictured feels best to you—with hands clasping your legs behind your knees or arms outstretched in front of you. Stay in the pose as long as you want, and breathe. See if you can hold for five or more breaths.

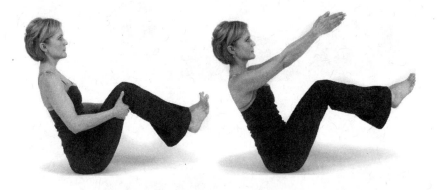

Chakra 4

- **Purpose:** To accept your emotions and your innate goodness and to receive divine intervention.

- **Mantra:** "I feel."

- Begin by reading or chanting **"I feel."**

- **Intention:** Work with your arms and your heart to reach out and receive.

Select one or more of the following poses for your practice.

Heart-Opening Flow

Kneel with your knees together; place a folded blanket under them if needed. Follow the movements of the arms demonstrated in the photos. Repeat the arm flow a few times. Breathe into and out from your heart center. Let your heart feel receptive.

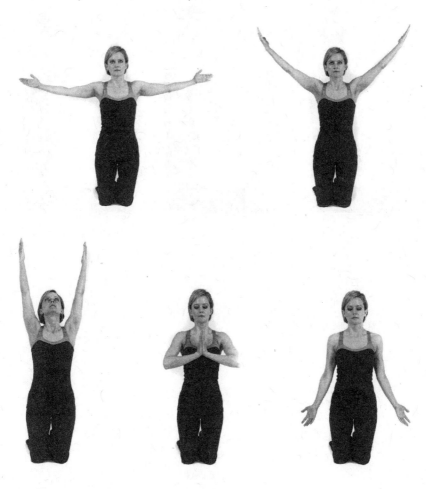

Chest-Opening Pose

Place your knees on the mat. Clasp your hands behind your back. Lift your hands as you inhale and lower your hands as you exhale. Be gentle; these are small movements. Repeat two or three times.

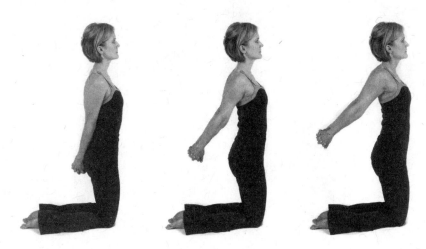

Camel Pose

Place your knees on the mat. Put your hands on your sacrum, the flat triangle-shaped bone in your lower back. If you have shoulder or neck issues, keep your head forward as depicted in the photo at left. Gently lift your chest as you lean back. Stay in your comfort zone so that you breathe easily.

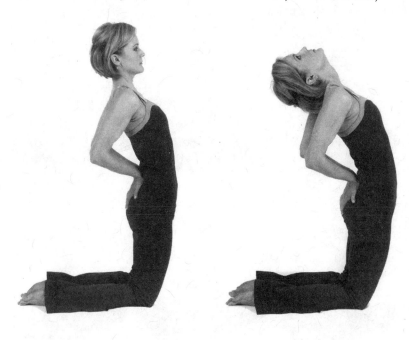

Chakra 5

- **Purpose:** To speak truthfully, express your heart, and stand up for justice.

- **Mantra:** "I express."

- Begin by reading or chanting **"I express."**

- **Intention:** Loosen your shoulders and neck, then sing, pray, or state a personal truth.

Chin Rolls

Sit comfortably. Relax your shoulders and rest your hands on your legs. Tuck your chin toward your chest. Roll your chin to the right side, back to center, and then over to the left side. Breathe in as you move toward your shoulders and breathe out as you move your chin toward your chest. Repeat a few times.

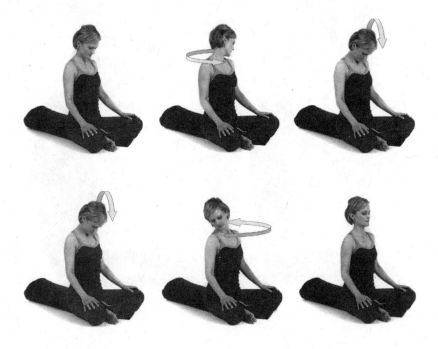

Metta **Prayer Pose**

Sit comfortably. Look straight ahead. Use your voice to sing or recite a song, **Metta** Prayer (introduced in chapter one), a scripture, or any prayer that you prefer.

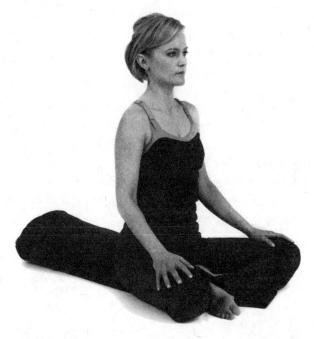

Chakra 6

- **Purpose:** To discern truth from non-truth and to access inner guidance and knowing.

- **Mantra:** "I know."

- Begin by reading or chanting **"I know."**

- **Intention:** Practice witnessing during longer holds, cultivating a quiet mind and deep listening.

After completing the seated spinal rotation, you may choose to do one or both of the eye practices.

Seated Spinal Rotation and Breath-Retention Practice

Before you begin, read this full description so that once you have reached your comfort zone in the pose you can remain there and concentrate solely on your practice. Sitting comfortably, rotate your spine to your right side. If possible, breathe in through your nose while you silently count to four. Then hold your breath for four counts. Then breathe out through your nose for eight counts. When you exhale, release your breath slowly so that you can exhale for the duration of the count. (But if you run out of breath and need to inhale, do so.) Then breathe in and repeat. If comfortable, on the third round, breathe in for four counts, hold your breath for seven, and breathe out for eight counts. Relax your breathing. Stay in the pose for a few more seconds, observing your breath and the physical sensations of stretching.

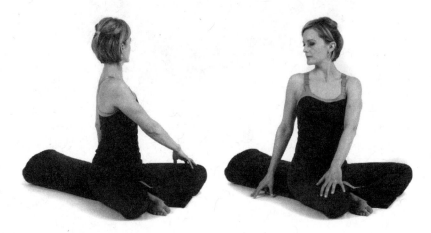

Rotate your spine to your left side and repeat the breath-retention practice followed by a few seconds of observing breath and physical sensations.

Eye Movements

Remain seated. Practice the eye movements as shown in the photo. First move your eyes up and down four times. Then move your eyes from side to side four times. Move comfortably and slowly. Conclude by gazing softly at the floor in front of you.

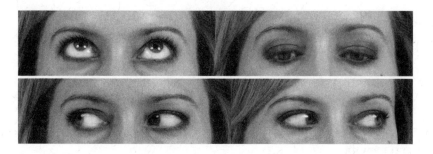

Eye Palming

Warm your hands by rubbing them together then place your cupped palms over your eyes with your fingers resting comfortably above your eyebrows. Focus your attention first on your eyebrows and then move your attention two inches into your brain behind and slightly above your eyebrows. Breathe into and out from this area in your brain. Stay in this pose for a few minutes, breathing quietly.

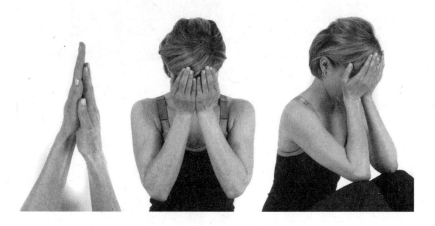

Chakra 7

- **Purpose:** To experience profound connection with ultimate reality.

- **Mantra:** "I am."

- Begin by reading or chanting **"I am."**

- **Intention:** Rest with top of forehead on floor, in a state of devotional surrender.

Select one of the two pictured poses. Alternatively, do one pose and then the other.

Child's Pose

In the pose of a child, let your cheek lie against the floor or a blanket. Rest comfortably in this pose for three or more minutes.

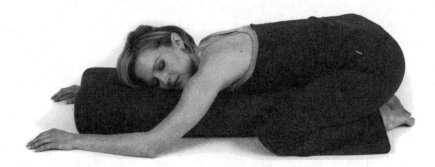

Yoga Mudra Pose

In yoga mudra pose, let the top of your forehead rest on the floor, folded blanket, or bolster. Choose the arm position that feels most appropriate. Rest comfortably in this pose for three or more minutes.

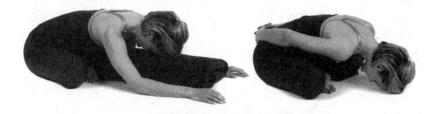

Final Resting Pose

End your practice in final resting pose, also called **shavasana**. Lie flat on your back. Allow your legs to gently fall out to the sides with feet hip-width apart or more. Allow your arms to relax a few inches beyond the sides of your torso, palms facing upward. If you have lower-back discomfort, place a folded blanket under your knees. Alternatively, rest on your stomach and support your head with your folded arms. Over time, as you feel able, rest on your back. Rest here for six to fifteen minutes, letting your entire being integrate the benefits of your practice.

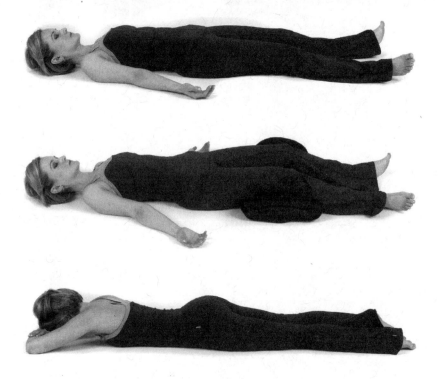

In Summary

Traumas—big and small, old and new—are imprinted in muscles as well as your nervous system. Doing a well-designed practice of yoga poses works tension patterns out of muscles. It teaches your body how to relax, releases pent-up energy, and more.

Mind, body, and spirit exist as a unit, and emotions represent their interactions. As such, emotions are body-mind experiences that are felt as energy. In the yoga philosophy, humans are fundamentally energy, and chakras are energy vortexes through which you take in, experience, and manifest life energy. Trauma gets lodged in these energy centers, resulting in imbalance. When they remain imbalanced trauma lives on. Balancing your energy centers results in profound healing.

A regular practice of a series of physical poses is far more than just a workout. Done faithfully, with reverence and a little knowledge, yoga yokes together body, mind, and spirit. Each day that you go to your mat, you submit to its healing power. Like a warm spring rain, a well-designed yoga practice melts away trauma that is frozen in your muscles and nervous system, allowing emotional and spiritual energy to flow freely through you.

chapter 5

paying attention to life in the present moment

the central message of this chapter is: the more you pay atten-tion, the happier you are. Learning to pay attention intentionally is important for everyone. However, when you have a history of trauma, learning to pay attention to what you want to pay attention to is also tremendously healing. In this chapter you'll learn what trauma does to attention and how being selective about what you pay attention to gives you new life.

We begin by reviewing what attention is and how it functions. We continue by discussing the two basic types of attention and the relationships between attention and memory and attention and thoughts. Next we discuss the significant effects, including decreas-ing your awareness of the present moment, that trauma has on attention. Then we explore how paying attention intentionally dis-solves the lingering effects of trauma. Finally, we teach easy, focused present-moment practices that teach you to pay attention fully to what is going on in the here and now.

In brief, trauma has a dramatic effect on your attention. It causes you to pay attention to some things and to disregard other things. For example, let's say that your house was broken into one night as you slept. Even after installing a house alarm system, when you settle into bed you might find yourself paying attention to house sounds rather than the pleasant physical sensations of being curled up under the covers. As a result, you feel afraid rather than safe even when there is no immediate threat.

Also, in the midst of traumatic incidents you generally do not focus on what is unbearable, such as intense pain. During such times you are only partially aware. You may know what is going on around you but not what you are experiencing inside your body. This unconscious response is adaptive at the time. But over time, being only partially aware can become habitual and feel normal, as though it is simply the way you are. As a result, you remain aware of some things, but not others. You may be highly aware of your inner life and less aware of what is going on around you, or it can be the other way around—you may be acutely aware of what is going on around you and less aware of bodily sensations and emotions. This pattern of partial awareness prevents full recovery from trauma. It also robs you of experiencing life in all its richness.

Present-moment focus practices train you to be more aware of what you are doing when you are doing it. While practicing, you learn to pay attention on purpose and you also decrease the habits of partial awareness and paying attention primarily to distressing thoughts or other stimuli, such as house sounds. They also show you how connected you are to each passing moment. These practices are comforting and enjoyable and reveal three things:

1. You are generally happier when you are focused on life in the present moment.

2. Much unhappiness is created by habitual patterns of partial attention and focusing on the negative.

3. You have choice about what you pay attention to.

About Attention

As a species we are unsurpassed in our capacity to focus on what we choose, thanks to the most recently evolved region of the human brain, the frontal lobes. With training you can be selective about what you pay attention to. You can learn to focus on things that make you happy rather than unintentionally paying attention to thoughts and experiences that perpetuate suffering. The following information about attention lays the groundwork for you to be able to focus on your own well-being and the goodness of life.

There are two basic kinds of attention. One, called *bottom-up*, is choiceless attention. The more primitive parts of the brain—the brain stem and the limbic system (discussed in chapter three)—are responsible for ensuring the survival of your physical body. If they perceive something threatening, they commandeer your attention. You instantly focus on whatever is threatening and, for the moment, you forget whatever else you were paying attention to.

Bottom-up attention is hardwired and happens automatically. In the same reflexive way that you jerk your hand away from a heated iron, you look in the direction of a sharp sound. For example, not long ago, Rick heard a loud knocking coming from the front of the house. Startled, he hurriedly rushed to investigate and found a determined woodpecker pecking on the side of the house. After his thinking brain reported that nothing was wrong he felt amused. However, for the brief interlude, he was choicelessly distracted from his computer work.

The second kind of attention, called *top-down*, involves choice. The part of your brain above your eyebrows, the prefrontal lobes, performs this function. Your frontal lobes are engaged when you intentionally focus, such as when you decide to put down the newspaper and pay attention to what your child is saying. Unlike bottom-up attention, top-down attention is trainable. You can learn to pay attention on purpose.

Bottom-up attention takes precedence over top-down attention. Preserving your life is top priority, so your brain is continuously alert to clues of danger. As you probably know, seeing a flame flare in the toaster distracts you from just about anything else you were focused on. However, your brain isn't just on the lookout for danger in your outer world. It also scans for signs of impending danger in your inner world of thoughts, sensations, and emotions. The pain of burning your finger on a toaster momentarily takes your full attention. Frightening thoughts distract your attention just as powerfully as physical pain. For example, the panicky thought "something's wrong; something's wrong" is going to make it next to impossible for you to focus on anything else.

Fortunately, you can train yourself to recognize what you are paying attention to and then change your focus when it's healing or wise to do so. You cannot prevent bottom-up attention from happening, nor do you want to. It is too important for your survival. However, a few moments after checking out the knocking sound or doing whatever you need to do to determine that you and your family are safe, you can engage top-down attention.

Often, it is not danger in your outer world but your body's fear response or fear-producing thoughts that captures bottom-up attention. When that is the case, as soon as you realize what is going on you can learn to redirect your attention to something that steadies and reassures you. The point is that you do not have to suffer from thoughts and sensations that perpetuate trauma.

The Power of Paying Attention

The Yoga Sutras of Patanjali state that learning to pay attention is central to yoga. T. K. V. Desikachar (1995, 149) translates sutra 1.2 as saying, "Yoga is the ability to direct the mind exclusively toward any object and sustain that direction without any distraction." Implied in this sutra is choice. You have choice about what you focus on. In fact, you may not realize just how much choice you actually have. Yet, to a large degree, what you pay attention to determines your experience.

Following is an example of focusing on safety rather than danger. A few years ago we drove on a winding gravel road that had been cut into the side of a mountain. The road was unnervingly close to the sheer drop-off. Focusing on the edge of the narrow road made Rick, who was driving, anxious. The only way to safely drive was to look directly at the road ahead. Although the ride was a tense one, especially where the road had partially eroded away, careful concentration made it possible. In a similar manner, your healing depends upon your learning to pay attention in ways that keep you safe and moving forward in your healing.

What You Can Pay Attention to and What Limits Attention

You can only pay attention to what is occurring in the present moment. Your present moment is made up of what is happening in your inner world of thoughts, emotions, and sensations and what is going on in the immediate environment around you. (When your attention is absorbed in thoughts about the past or the future, you are paying attention to the subject matter of thoughts. Unaware that you are producing the thoughts, you take the contents of your thoughts to be reality. The act of thinking itself only arises in real time.)

Certainly things go on around and within you that escape your attention. Intensely focusing on something, such as a canyon far below, decreases your ability to focus elsewhere, such as on the bumpy road in front of you. Second, your capacity to pay attention may not be highly developed, meaning that you have not been trained to select and sustain focus. Third, trauma can significantly impair your capacity to pay attention on purpose.

The Effects of Trauma on Attention

Life-threatening and highly stressful events cause your more primitive brain centers (brain stem and limbic system) to kick into high gear as they attempt to protect you. As a result, blood flow to your prefrontal lobe, the brain region that pays attention on purpose, is diminished. Your ability to concentrate and make sense of it all is not restored until blood flow to your prefrontal lobes increases again, which happens once you are out of harm's way and calmer. However, even after you are safe, you do not become calm until the nervous system's fight-flight-or-freeze responses are discharged.

(Knowing this, you can choose to run in place or vigorously shake your hands to release this pent-up energy.)

If your nervous system stays amped up, your attention may be more bottom-up than top-down. For instance, if you are the type who is easily startled or hypervigilant, your attention is like a sentry on the lookout for danger, at least in some situations. For instance, some people become hyperaware of how their spouses look at other potential sexual partners. At parties they are distracted from their own conversations because they are on guard, looking for cues of possible betrayal. As disturbing as this preoccupation is, and in spite of wishing to focus elsewhere, their attention is fixated on their partner's actions. You can't blame your attention for this behavior—it is just doing its job. However, this preoccupation causes suffering.

Additionally, a hallmark response to trauma is feeling disconnected from what is going on. Called *dissociation*, this reaction happens when threatening circumstances overwhelm your ability to cope. When the experience is too frightening, painful, frequent, or awful your nervous system goes into protective mode, possibly causing you to feel numb. If the trauma feels (or is) life threatening, you may experience yourself as being outside of your body as an onlooker to what is happening. While out-of-body occurrences are a benevolent response of the nervous system, they also bring to mind the yogic inquiry "Who am I?" Out-of-body experiences verify that consciousness is not confined to the body.

Attention and Dissociation

Dissociation is not knowing, at least in part, what you are experiencing and/or what is going on around you. It is as if your nervous system is saying, "I'll let you be aware of this but not that." Dissociation can take several forms, such as blunting physical sensations so that you do not feel pain or causing events around you to feel surreal or dreamlike. It can also block out memories and emotions so that you do not face what is too overwhelming, which is why, all these years later, Mary cannot remember the exact date in August of her sister's sudden death.

For a more detailed example of dissociation, we go to Rick. He was in a serious airplane accident (which we further discuss in chapter six) along with his flight instructor, Mark. It took the rescue team five hours to get them to the hospital, where Mary was waiting. While the medical staff worked on Rick, Mark, who had sustained only minor injuries, told Mary the story of the terrifying crash in minute detail. He had dried blood streaks on his face but showed no emotion—his body didn't even tremble during the retelling. His overstressed nervous system had walled off pain and emotional distress. Initially, in a state of shock, this disconnect had helped him function. Not being distracted by intense discomfort, he had been able to radio for help and pull Rick from the wreckage to protect him should the plane catch on fire. However, shock transitioned into ongoing disconnect. He remained walled off from his emotions for some time, and this prevented Mark from feeling grief and regret for many months.

As the example suggests, memories of traumatic events can have missing pieces. Disconnect can take several forms, such as remembering some aspects of what happened but not other aspects. Or remembering events but not the emotions. Alternatively, you may remember scenes, sounds, smells, or body sensations but not what actually happened. One way or another, memory is only partial and is not totally integrated.

But gradually, over time, integrated memories are possible. Let's continue with our example. Six months after the accident, we had a lengthy conversation about the ill-fated flight with Mark and his wife. It turned into an intellectual discussion during which Mark talked about if or how he could have prevented the crash. Afterward, we watched a triumphant video clip of a British woman singing on a talent show. Tears streamed from Mark's eyes as he listened to the beautiful song. It was not until another conversation a year later that Mark realized that his tears that night, triggered by the emotional song, had expressed grief and regret about the accident. In making that association his memory became more integrated.

With integrated memories you can recall the actual event, including what you saw, heard, smelled, tasted, and touched. You can also recall what it was like for you, including associated emotions and physical sensations. For instance, in a positive memory of a wedding, you recall the setting, the sounds of the music, the sweaty delight of dancing, the sweet taste of wedding cake, and the shared joy. It is a complete body-mind experience.

Attention and Addiction

The aftermath of trauma is also associated with addictions. If you have ever eaten a second piece of cake, just for the comfort of it, or drank a glass of wine to relax, you can appreciate how easy it is to overuse food, drugs, and alcohol in the aftermath of trauma. All three can dull your consciousness to the extent that it is like you are half asleep, which makes paying attention next to impossible. They also temporarily soothe an amped-up nervous system, as this next example demonstrates.

Susan is a young woman who encountered an intruder as he walked into her kitchen from the garage door. Fortunately, he turned and ran off. However, Susan became afraid to sleep for fear that she would not hear him if he returned again. Increasingly exhausted and anxious, she developed an evening martini habit to numb fear so she could get some rest. Being intoxicated helped her get through the night but did not help her heal from the trauma. Two years later, after her mood dangerously plummeted, she sought out professional therapy to help her on her path to recovery. Attempting to deal with trauma by drugging oneself into a slump, eating oneself into a state of inertia, or drinking oneself into a haze makes matters worse, as Susan discovered.

127

Addictions are progressive and result in tragedy. Fortunately, you have choice and you can be in recovery. If you have a serious addiction, search out a treatment program and become involved with a twelve-step program, such as Alcoholics Anonymous, Narcotics Anonymous, or Overeaters Anonymous.

Attention and Thoughts

Nothing captures your attention as frequently as thoughts do. As a result, you, and just about everyone else, spend a lot of time focusing on thoughts. In an interesting study, Matthew Killingsworth and Paul Gilbert (2010) reported that people spend nearly half of their waking hours paying attention to thoughts rather than to what is happening. With so much attention consumed by thoughts, you inevitably miss out on what is going on inside and around you. That is a lot of time lost and a lot of life missed out on.

When your attention wanders off in thoughts you are less aware of life as it arises. Your present-moment experience, however real it feels, is contrived. Produced by thoughts, your experience may be quite disconnected from what is going on around you. In effect, you are creating a daydream—only you do not know it is a daydream. You think that it is real. The contents of thoughts feel real due to the intimacy they have with physical sensations and emotions. Remember: mind and body live as one. When your attention is absorbed in evocative thoughts, the moment feels as real as night dreams do. And often, especially when it comes to thoughts about painful things that have happened, diverting your attention away from them is as relieving as waking up out of a bad dream at night.

Unfortunately, unpleasant thoughts that replay trauma capture your attention almost as predictably as bread burning in the toaster does. Bear in mind that the parts of your brain that are designed to help you survive dangerous situations have a built-in partiality to noticing pain-producing, negative thoughts. Fortunately, you can unplug from such thoughts as quickly as you can pull an appliance cord out of the electrical socket. All it takes is recognizing what is happening and focusing your attention elsewhere.

Following is a statement you can utter to refocus your attention away from pain-producing thoughts: "I am not going to think about all that stuff right now and get upset." After making such a comment, get up and do something else and be mindful of what you are doing. There is a time and place to deal with difficulties. (We are not suggesting denial or avoidance.) However, just before going to bed, at wedding receptions, or during holiday gatherings are not the best times to address unresolved trauma. Also, there is little benefit in wallowing in thoughts about painful memories.

Attention and Memory

You have two types of memory: explicit and implicit. *Explicit memory* is the ability to recall names, numbers, people, and events. This kind of information is not permanently imprinted in your brain, and you can easily forget such data as old addresses, phone numbers, or airline flight numbers when you no longer have use for them. *Implicit memory* pertains to emotions, motor skills (riding a bicycle), and conditioned sensory motor responses (your foot tapping when you hear a favorite song). Implicit memory is relatively permanent. Even if you have not ridden a bicycle for decades, you could get on one and, after a little wobbling, find your balance. Explicit memories imprinted with intense emotions are also seared into your implicit memory and may pop into awareness when triggered by similar sensory experiences. That is why, while walking down a hospital corridor to visit a friend, the sounds and smells may cause you to unexpectedly recall an agonizing emergency room visit you made many years ago.

Procedural memory, a subset of implicit memory, pertains to learning how to do things and usually comes about as the result of ongoing practice. For example, becoming an impressive card shuffler is the result of many hours of practice and several decks of cards. However, procedural memory does not always rely on repetition. Your body is conditioned quickly in response to life-threatening trauma. According to Robert Scaer (2005), whatever your body does in response to threat—such as your hand flying up to cover your face—is burned into permanent procedural memory. In response to future perceived threat, your brain will automatically activate the same survival skill that it learned previously.

For example, while driving on an expressway a decade ago, Mary's car was rear-ended by a honking van that had no brakes. She attempted to change lanes, but there was no opening in the traffic. Just before impact, she automatically hunched up her shoulders and dropped her chin down toward her chest. Even though it was a noninjury accident, for several months following the incident her body, reacting to procedural memory, prepared for impact from braking cars behind her even when there was no threat, such as when Mary was stopped at a red light. To this day her shoulders hunch slightly when she prepares to move into another lane.

Whatever your body has done to survive, that behavior goes into procedural memory. And procedural memory can also respond to internal cues (such as thoughts) of a threat that does not exist in the present moment. For Mary, just thinking about driving in rush-hour traffic in a major city causes tension in her shoulders. That's the power of procedural memory.

Present-Moment Concentration Practices

Present-moment concentration practices are top-down ways of paying attention. As a practice, they consist of selecting something to focus on, other than thoughts, and then paying attention to what you have chosen. Let your attention be alert, yet relaxed, so that you feel neither physically nor mentally tense. Examples of what to focus on include a specific physical sensation (feeling the bottoms of your feet touching the floor) or a sensory input (listening to beautiful violin music). As you are about to discover, focusing, then keeping your attention focused, on something as ordinary as the sensation of your hands resting on your lap feels quite nice, diverts attention away from disturbing thoughts, and has a surprisingly calming effect.

These practices are pleasant and teach you about the richness of ordinary life. To say it simply, trauma and its aftermath feel awful; but to discover again, or perhaps for the first time, that life is enjoyable is a wonderful feat. Learning to pay attention to what is happening in the present moment gives you your life back.

Stabilizing Body Scan

Doing a simple body scan is very grounding. This is a go-to practice for when you feel like you are on the verge of losing emotional control. This firm but loving practice takes your attention away from distress and plants it in your feet and hips. When your attention is rooted in the lower half of your physical body you feel stable, solid. Your nervous system relaxes and your thinking mind becomes quiet. Fortunately, thoughts, when not paid attention to, tend to drift away, like dandelion seed heads in the wind. They may blow back in the next moment, but with your attention stabilized in your hips, you do not give them much attention. With little to attach to, your thoughts are much more likely to float on by.

Read through the body-scan instructions slowly and practice while you read.

INSTRUCTIONS FOR DOING A BODY SCAN

While seated, place both feet squarely on the floor. Notice your right foot and your left foot planted on the floor. Feel the inside and outside of each foot placed on the floor. Next, move your attention up both lower legs, to your knees. Now direct your attention up to your hips in the chair. Feel the weight of gravity pressing both hips down. Move your awareness up your spine, feeling your shoulders resting on the back of the chair. Now direct your attention back down to your hips. Steadily focus on the sensations of your hips touching the seat. Keep your attention on your hips. Notice that you can continue to read while softly focusing on your hips. Maintaining this focus prevents you from being easily distracted.

The Practice of Floor Gazing

Vision orients you to your external surroundings so that you know where you are and what is going on around you. Interestingly, vision has a direct line to your limbic system so that it can quickly scan incoming images to assess for possible danger. That is why you may become hypervigilant when you are really frightened. Hypervigilance is automatically (not intentionally) keeping a watchful eye on your immediate surroundings. Scanning intensely, you look for the danger that your body says is present, even when nothing threatening is happening.

The practice of intentional steady gazing can soothe your nerves and remind you that you are in a safe place. Since vision is so orienting, softly focusing at a specific area, preferably on something that is not moving, can really tamp down your body's fear response. And, with very few exceptions, the floor in front of you is motionless and predictable.

Gazing at the floor in front of you keeps you focused on where you are. Also, if you are in a safe place, focusing on the floor reminds you of that, as this next example illustrates. Rebecca came to Mary's office for help in getting out of an abusive relationship. Beaten down mentally and physically, she did not see a way out. She was terrified, concerned that her boyfriend would hunt her down and kill her. Rebecca practiced floor gazing, sitting in the office, until her nervous system recognized it as a safe space. Rebecca then took the practice out into her life. Floor gazing helped her discern safe places, like the grocery store, from dangerous ones, like her home during times when her boyfriend was drinking beer. After some time she was able to go to classes at a domestic-violence intervention program and attend church services. She also used floor gazing to steady herself when she was at home, especially when her boyfriend was out of the house. Eventually, she purchased and moved into a home in a nearby community. Once she was in a non-harmful environment, she was no longer attracted to floor gazing as a practice. It had served her well and it was time to move on.

INSTRUCTIONS FOR FLOOR GAZING

While seated in a comfortable position, look at the floor directly in front of you. Study it. Notice color variations, patterns, intersections, straight lines, curving lines, dirt, texture, stains. Move your eyes slightly to gaze a little farther away. Notice where furniture touches the floor, where the floor and wall meet, if in your line of vision. Continue to look at the floor. Let your eyes be soft and relaxed, let your eyes blink comfortably as you focus. Notice that as you gaze, your mind quiets and your body relaxes.

Floor gazing and body scans are "come to your rescue" stabilizing practices for you to do when you are really upset.

Gazing at a Sacred Symbol

This practice is an extension of gazing meditation and is a way to be reminded of the sacred throughout the day.

To do this practice, first intentionally place objects in your home and work environment that symbolize what is precious or most sacred to you, for instance: candle flames that fill you with a sense of eternal light, flowers that fill you with beauty, pictures of loved ones that fill your heart with love. Place the object(s) in plain view so that it is easily accessible, preferably in an area where you spend a lot of your time.

Second, take the time, off and on throughout the day, to pause and pay attention to your sacred symbols. Pause long enough to feel the qualities that they represent arise within you. The gazing becomes contemplative as the thoughts and emotions associated with the object are embedded into your psyche.

This lovely practice not only cultivates one-pointed attention, it settles your mind, fills it with meaning, and makes you aware of the eternal. For example, in her office Mary has placed photos of beloved dogs who have died. Photos of Bubba, Star Girl, and Gracie are positioned where she can easily see them. They remind her that life in physical form is precious and transitory. "After a momentary glance at their pictures, I relax and my mind quiets," says Mary. "Then I sense the preciousness of the moment, which evaporates my tendency to feel pressed for time. These cherished pets remind me that life does not need for me to rush around, at least not most of the time."

You can also select other sensory representations of the sacred to focus on. You may like the smell of burning incense or the sound of an uplifting song. Rick frequently strikes a singing bowl bell that sits conveniently on a table he passes by when he walks into the kitchen. The sound of the bell takes him from preoccupation with detail to awareness of spaciousness. "Following the sound into silence takes me into inner stillness, where I feel peaceful and content," says Rick. "My psyche requires a daily diet of simple pleasures to quiet the internal critical voices that press for productivity and focus on what isn't right. Over the years, listening to the bell, and even watching birds outdoors, has weakened my habit of feeling irritable."

INSTRUCTIONS FOR SACRED SYMBOL GAZING

Give yourself a few minutes, a time-out from your activities. Stand or sit within a few feet of your sacred object so that you can easily look at it. Let your attention become absorbed in the symbol. Sense the energy that is represented by the symbol and let yourself respond emotionally. Alternatively, when walking by your sacred symbol, intentionally linger long enough to soak in its energy and meaning.

Paying Attention to Your Breath

Breath, ever available, is a great focal point for the practice of paying attention on purpose, anywhere, anytime. All that you need in order to be mindful of your breath is making the choice to do so. Choosing requires intentionality and also cultivates intentionality. Therefore, frequently taking a moment to focus on breathing helps you to become more intentional in general. Additionally, practicing paying attention to breathing when you are not upset makes it easier to focus on breathing when you are upset.

Paying attention to breathing is also a quiet way to be with yourself. When you focus on breathing you have a momentary reprieve from thinking. You literally get to feel yourself beneath the superficiality of your busy mind. And since breathing only occurs in the present moment, concentrating on breathing in and out brings you right into the middle of the present moment. You are here and now.

You can take a breathing break any time you want to. It does not take much time and it is a temporary respite from your usual preoccupation with tasks, habits, and thinking. It is beneficial to practice breath awareness when doing routine tasks that do not require intense focus, such as unloading the dishwasher. Although it is easy to perform mundane chores mechanically, doing so causes you to lose connection with the background sense of aliveness. Focusing on breath, on the other hand, reconnects you to an underlying experience of aliveness. That is why you feel real and not mechanical when you pay attention to breathing while putting away dishes, putting up groceries, or putting on your shoes.

Another benefit of focusing on breath, with its quiet sounds and subtle sensations, is that it sensitizes you to inner stillness. In the moment of tuning in to breathing, you connect to something more fundamental to who you are than thoughts and emotions. You could say that being aware of breathing helps you to reconnect with you inner self. No wonder taking a breather is so refreshing and fulfilling.

INSTRUCTIONS FOR PAYING ATTENTION TO BREATHING

Wherever you are, whatever you are doing, pause and notice that you are breathing in and out. Focus your attention on one full inhalation and one full exhalation. Now notice a couple more breaths.

Select a routine activity, such as locking the door at night or turning on the coffee pot in the morning. Write "Breathe" on a sticky note and attach it to your doorknob or coffeepot so that you have a reminder to pay attention to breathing while you perform the simple task.

Paying Attention to Eating Practice

Many of us eat without paying attention to eating. When you eat while being distracted or spaced out, you forgo the experience of eating, at least partially. Your mouth is chewing, but you are not completely there. As a result, you miss out on the full flavor and texture of your food. Eating absentmindedly is a specific experience of not being aware of the richness of ordinary life. In general, when life does not seem vivid or vibrant you are likely to feel bored and dissatisfied. Something as simple as paying attention to the experience of eating can bring vitality back into mealtime, because eating is such a strong sensory experience. And the more experiences you have of ordinary life being interesting the more contented you are.

If you are significantly overweight or have unhealthy eating habits that put your health at risk, we sincerely encourage you to do the enjoyable, daily eating practice we present shortly. This brief practice is most healing because it is an experience of mindful eating. Doing the practice frequently interrupts unhealthy eating habits and cultivates healthy ones. And, as you are about to find out, the practice is surprisingly easy to do.

Overeating is often associated with trauma, and eating disorders are complex. Entire books are written on this subject alone. The eating practice we outline is a very helpful component of healing, though it may be insufficient to heal a distressed relationship with food. If this is your case, do the practice daily but take a more comprehensive approach to recovery. Work with a team that includes a physician, a nutritionist, a counselor, and a support group. You and your health matter, so take appropriate steps to get the help you need.

The exercise that follows draws on the principles of a yoga practice called *pratyahara*, which means "withdrawal of the senses." It is a practice of closing your eyes and plugging your ears so that you do not see and/or hear. This practice helps you focus on inner sensations and is a way of shutting the world out. In the eating practice below, you may want to experiment with chewing with your eyes closed. Many people find that this enhances the experience and easily slows down chewing to a comfortable, optimal pace. If you tend to gobble your food, closing your eyes while doing this eating practice may be a rewarding option for you.

Also, if you are a fast eater, here is a tip: do not begin this brief practice when you are really hungry; wait until you have eaten part of your meal or snack so that you can enjoy the practice.

INSTRUCTIONS FOR PAYING ATTENTION TO EATING

This practice could be named "Eat and know that you are eating," since it consists of concentrating on biting, chewing, and swallowing.

This can be a brief practice—you do not have to do this during an entire meal. Decide on the length of your practice, but go easy on yourself. Select just a minute or two, especially if you are new to this exercise.

Sit down and heed these three instructions:

1. Refrain from multitasking. Only eat.

2. Place your eating utensil on your plate or napkin between bites.

3. Pay attention to biting, chewing, and swallowing.

Focus on the food going into your mouth, on chewing, on saliva moistening your mouth, on swallowing. It is as simple as that. When your formal practice is over, continue eating and enjoy the rest of your meal.

You may choose to do this exercise during part of a meal or while eating a snack such as a piece of fruit or a handful of nuts. You may also want to close your eyes during part or all of the practice.

Paying Attention to Walking Practice

The practice of mindful walking is recognized as coming from the Buddhist tradition. Since it is such a great way to practice paying attention to what you are doing, we include it here.

Walking occurs as a result of procedural memory. After you learned how to walk as a toddler, your unconscious memory took over and began doing the walking for you. Since you no longer have to think about placing one foot in the front of the other, it is easy to walk and think about anything and everything but walking. But when your attention is lost in the contents of thoughts, you are not as aware of what your body is doing and where it is at. Your body is in one place and you and your thoughts are somewhere else. That disconnect detracts from your sense of aliveness.

Since walking is associated with procedural memory, you can walk when you are sleepy or somewhat drugged. You can also walk in a partial state of dissociation, barely feeling the physical sensations of walking. And you can walk as a matter of habit and hardly know that you are walking, just because it is so familiar. But when you pay attention to one foot and then the other foot moving on the sidewalk, you are aware of where you are and what you are doing. If you tend to feel spacey or disconnected, a focused walking practice might not only be enjoyable, it may also be a healing experience of realizing that you are in your body and you are safe. Additionally, undertaking a walking meditation is a relieving alternative for those times when you feel too emotionally agitated for sitting meditation.

There is nothing wrong with taking a walk to do some serious thinking. That said, rather than walking and mulling things over it may be really beneficial to just walk and pay attention to walking. When you focus on walking, your thinking mind rests, making it more possible for you to hear the answers that reflect deeper wisdom.

You can practice walking any time you are up and moving. However, paying attention to walking is more enjoyable when you like where you are. Zen master Thich Nhat Hanh (2009) teaches that with each step you take you arrive into the present moment. Therefore it makes good sense to arrive into a pleasant moment.

INSTRUCTIONS FOR PAYING ATTENTION TO WALKING

Wear clothes and shoes that allow your body to be comfortable. Approach walking with curiosity, as though it were a fresh and new experience, which it is. After all, you have never taken this step before so pay attention to it. Keep a soft focus on the sensation of striding forward, heel to toe, heel to toe. Walk slowly with an easy gait so that your balance feels natural.

Select a short route and a time of day that appeal to you. We recommend a nearby outdoor course, such as a path around a tree in the backyard. Mindful walking does not have to be time consuming. Start with a few minutes, and then add more as you like. Go at about the same time each day so that you get into a routine.

You may also designate a routine task, such as picking up the morning newspaper from the driveway, as your practice time. Indoor routes, such as walking from the living room to the kitchen or from one wall to the opposite wall of a room for a brief period of time, work equally well.

Summary

You have two kinds of attention. Bottom-up attention is concerned with your survival. The other, top-down attention, is responsible for concentration, intentionality, and follow-through. These two types of attention work together to protect you and to help you develop skills and enjoy life. However, trauma disrupts your nervous system, causing it to perceive threat when there is none, which in turn inhibits your ability to pay attention on purpose. Additionally, trauma can cause you to numb out in a variety of ways. You cannot pay attention to what you are not aware of.

Concentrating on ordinary experiences, such as the sensations of your hips in the chair, breathing, eating, and walking, teaches you to focus on what is going on in and around you, which is the opposite of acting mechanically and feeling numb. These practices teach you how to stay in the moment rather than running away into the contents of thoughts. Finally, they help you discover, perhaps for the first time, the joy and comfort of feeling alive in ordinary life.

chapter 6

dealing with physical
and emotional pain

the effects of trauma can be long lived due to the physical and emotional pain that often follows in its aftermath. In the course of a lifetime most people experience a life-changing trauma or pain, as they are very common experiences. Yet each experience is unique, and you may feel alone in your suffering. It is also true that reading about how someone else got through a really tough time may help you feel less alone and give you ideas for dealing with your pain. Therefore, we open this chapter with Rick's story of trauma and pain.

Next we address the emotional ramifications of physical pain and explain how natural and inevitable they are. We do this as a gentle way to bring pain and suffering into the light of consciousness so that it can be recognized and lovingly tended to. Finally, we present yoga practices and meditations that bring healing and understanding to pain and suffering.

Rick's Story of Trauma

Rick's story of trauma began in May 2009, when he survived a near-fatal airplane crash. He had been flying with an instructor to practice recovery techniques for unusual flight altitudes. On their third maneuver they were unable to recover the airplane and crashed into a remote wooded area.

About an hour after the crash, a pilot who was flying an aircraft in the vicinity heard the radio distress call and notified the authorities. A rescue team was assembled. After hiking through the forest, they made their way to the accident site just as nightfall and a thunderstorm were upon them. The men carried Rick for more than a half mile on a stretcher to an all-terrain vehicle that took him to an ambulance.

At the hospital the ER surgeon put more than a hundred stitches in Rick's forearms and informed us that Rick had a broken shoulder and a broken ankle. The next morning the orthopedic surgeon said, "This is a very serious injury." He took Rick into surgery in an attempt to save his foot. A few hours later Rick came out of surgery with both arms wrapped in bandages, his right arm in a sling, and his right foot in a restraining boot. We opted to go home a couple of days later and use home health care nurses rather than stay in the hospital during recovery.

His Pain Trauma

Unrelenting pain, not the airplane crash itself, was the primary source of trauma for Rick. As he said, "After all, accidents happen." For fourteen months, morning after morning he was greeted by intense pain that stayed with him until sleep gave him a few hours of reprieve. The hardest part for him was not the moment-by-moment experience of pain but the recurring thoughts about not knowing if the pain would ever subside.

As a result, his equanimity depended upon his staying in moment-by-moment awareness. "The only way I got through those months was by focusing on the present moment, when I was able to," recalls Rick. "If only" thoughts about the past and "what if" thoughts about the future just brought more mental suffering. For example, when he drifted into thoughts like, "What if this pain never stops?" he had to breathe deeply and refocus by saying, "Stay here."

Finally, after six months of intense pain and not being able to bear weight on his immobilized right foot, physical therapy was ordered. Healed or not, the surgeon said that rehabilitating his very stiff foot could wait no longer. Therapy meant six more months of intense physical pain—like "someone pounding nails in my foot"— even with the use of powerful pain medication. His pain notably subsided after a simple surgery provided relief, and in July 2010 he took his last pain medication.

His mental haze, irritability, and sadness slowly subsided. Moderate pain remained, although it gradually decreased over time. In September 2010 Rick hiked for one mile on a mountain trail, fulfilling his desire to hike in the mountains—a goal that had kept him motivated to keep showing up for physical therapy. The following summer Rick completed a couple of four-mile mountain hikes.

Still, several times throughout the day, Rick holds and massages his foot. He is not pain-free—and there may be future surgeries—but he can take an evening walk in the nearby woods, tend to his work, focus on creative projects, and laugh and play again.

His Emotional Trauma

The second source of trauma was the betrayal of trust and competency Rick felt toward Mark, the flight instructor who was flying with Rick during the accident, because he had not closely monitored the flight for safety. Although highly trained and experienced, Mark instructed Rick to begin a stall procedure at an altitude too low to recover from. Fortunately, once Mark realized the impending danger, he took control of the airplane and his flight skills prevented the crash from being more serious than it was, saving both their lives.

Rick resumed flying after the accident. In 2011 he went through an intensive flight-training program that included flying with flight instructors for many hours. During flight lessons Rick was required to wear a view-limiting device that restricted his vision to just the aircraft instruments. Once again Rick's life depended upon the skill of the instructor. Although each instructor Rick flew with kept them safe, Rick experienced sweaty, breath-gripping, heart-pounding panic attacks. "My brain would just go blank," recalls Rick, "and I could not remember instructions or execute maneuvers that I had mentally rehearsed and practiced in the plane many times."

The emotional stress impeded Rick's progress. One flight instructor, apparently impatient with Rick's anxiety, became more critical in his teaching style. His sharp words, loud sighs, and critical remarks reminded Rick of his father's temperament. Memories of childhood trauma piled on top of recent trauma. When flying alone Rick's skills were flawless, but when he performed for his instructor he made several mistakes. Rick questioned his ability to pass his upcoming flight examination.

Rick recognized that what he was experiencing were responses to trauma. Putting his life in an instructor's hands terrified him, and being taught in an intimidating, unkind manner triggered a freeze response in him, just as it had decades earlier when he was a boy. Knowing that as an adult he has choice, Rick changed instructors and quickly completed his training with a man who was kind and reassuring. Shortly thereafter he demonstrated his competency to a flight examiner and passed his flight test.

Emotional Ramifications of Physical Pain

Healing and managing pain is a step-by-step, hour-by-hour journey that is like being in a precarious, unfamiliar land with no precise map to follow. If you have been there, you know that along the way you may encounter sleeplessness, misunderstandings about your pain, and a whole range of unexpected emotions. In truth, it is not an easy journey. However, the more you know about these emotions and how to lovingly take care of them, the less likely they are to intensify physical pain, overwhelm you, or discourage you so much that you give up on healing. Even though there is no precise roadmap for healing, you can get a sense of the terrain in this chapter, which will aid you in understanding emotions as they arise. The following insight may help.

Since your body's state of well-being is reflected in thoughts and emotions, it is natural that you experience emotional distress when you are in physical pain. Grief and irritability often accompany pain. To help you appreciate these and other emotions that are associated with pain, we are going to discuss pain and its ramifications.

Physical pain involves change and limitation, especially around mobility, pleasurable activities, interest in others, and daily routines. In the aftermath of physical injury, life shrinks, at least for a while. It can hurt too much to ride in a car, carry children, have sexual relations, haul groceries, go for a walk, sit in a chair, or do household chores. "Excruciating pain made my life small," says Rick. "For the first year and a half [after the plane crash] my life consisted of my foot, me, and sometimes Mary, in that order." Little else interested him during that period of agony and healing.

As you probably know, pain can be dull, throbbing, sharp, jolting, piercing, and attention grabbing. And, when the pain level is great, very few things can distract your attention from it. The smell of bread baking, the sight of the sun setting, and the sounds of children playing probably pass by unnoticed. This means that when pain is unrelenting, your mood is not lifted by pleasantries that you usually enjoy.

Then there is fear of pain. Wanting to escape from pain and to minimize it seem like normal human reactions to pain, reactions you truly understand if you have experienced intense pain. Also, ongoing pain may cause you to inadvertently back away from full recovery because rehabilitation often involves intense physical sensations. Having low tolerance for discomfort may cause you to underestimate your capacity to heal and even to retreat from therapies that could facilitate recovery. As Rick noted during his months in physical therapy, "I see why people resist a full course of physical therapy and settle for partial improvement. Your mind recoils from pain that seems unbearable."

If pain persists, over time you may become increasingly inactive, which causes your energy, mobility, and mood to decline. On the other hand, you may overestimate your capacity and injure yourself by performing tasks that your body is not able to do. That is emotionally upsetting because just when you think you are getting better you suffer a setback.

The Stigma of Chronic Pain

How you emotionally respond to pain is influenced by what your doctors, family, and culture at large think about chronic pain. First of all, pain is invisible. Since no one else can see or feel your pain, outsiders sometimes doubt its severity. Second, because there is stigma around chronic pain, people may wonder if you are simply weak or not motivated.

The National Institutes of Health reports that sixteen million Americans experience chronic pain and that chronic pain is the top cited reason for seeking medical care. Unfortunately, as Richard Besdine (2011) reports, health care providers, unavoidably subjected to prevailing social attitudes about pain, may perceive complaints of pain to be exaggerated, imagined, or inevitable. Many health care providers are undertrained in pain management and think that physical dependence on pain medications is addiction, which is not the case. Also, for many reasons, most doctors are considerably cautious about prescribing pain medications.

Rick's experience is not unusual. The health care provider who prescribed to Rick was cautious and regularly warned, after six months of usage, that this prescription may be the last. At the time, Rick's pain level was still very high. Worry about not having his pain managed caused Rick to underuse his medications in order to save a small supply in the event his request for a prescription was denied. Rick's need for pain management became a source of emotional strain for him, as it is for many.

Sleep Disturbance and Chronic Pain

Chronic and intense pain impacts sleep. When the house is dark and still, you are left alone with your inner life, including emotional, mental, and physical pain. Pain, now more noticeable, makes getting to sleep and staying asleep difficult. In a vicious cycle, pain begets sleep disturbance, and lack of sleep is clearly linked to depression, irritability, low energy, and muddled thinking. In fact, Vivien Burt (2004) found that one of the most commonly shared features of chronic pain, depression, and anxiety is sleep disturbance. Sleep deprivation is so closely linked to emotional trauma that we present practices that both promote sleep and help deal with sleeplessness.

Loss and Grief

The wounds of trauma and the aftermath of pain are simply heartbreaking. After a while, shock gives way to loss and loss gives way to grief. While your personal experience of loss is your own, the list of possible losses that go with trauma is long. You may experience loss of self-worth, loss of familiar ways of doing tasks, loss of financial stability, loss of living in a body that feels good and moves easily, loss of activity, loss of personal relationships, loss of trust, loss of dreams, loss of ordinary reference points (routines, what you wear, etc.), and more.

Loss of self-worth can be especially acute if pain causes you to be unable to work at home and/or on the job. The ability to contribute and be productive looms large in our societal attitudes about self-worth. Even though your worth cannot be reduced to what you do and the roles you play, these powerful beliefs can be a choke hold on self-esteem, a grip that you can only understand when such a loss happens to you.

Sometimes injury disfigures, prematurely ages, and/or causes changes in your body. You may feel like you have a different body, one that looks, feels, and functions in unfamiliar ways. Your body may have new aches and pains and in general feel uncomfortable. If your body hurts more and does less than it used to, you may well grieve for the body that was easier to live in.

Finally, with life-altering trauma, sooner or later you experience the loss of the hoped-for future. In all reality, you may not be able to fulfill old desires, at least not in the ways you once imagined. Letting go of unrealized dreams, no matter how big or dear, can be pure agony. One of Rick's losses is the ability to scamper up rugged mountain hiking trails. One day he mused, "With more pain and arthritis possible in the future, I am tempted to portion out my steps, in case I have a limited supply of them, so I can save some for hiking." In the next breath, after feeling the mixture of sadness and anxiety the thoughts produced, he whispered, "Stay here, stay here in this moment."

Grief is normal and inevitable but that does not mean it is easy. A little like childbirth, it rips and opens you as it works its way through your body, heart, and mind. The reality is that grief can seem intolerable at times as it waxes and wanes according to its own timeline. Fortunately, like Rick discovered, you only have to deal with grief one breath at a time—and over time it does subside. Grief is also a wise teacher that helps you to appreciate the exquisiteness of passing moments and become clear about what really matters to you.

Depression, anxiety, and irritability are often indistinguishable from grief and, in fact, they often arise simultaneously. Yet it helps to separate them in order to understand and identify them. So that you appreciate how closely related they are to pain we include some research and physiology in the following discussions.

Depression

There is a well-documented overlapping relationship between depression and chronic pain. Estimates vary, but researchers L. R.

Miller (2009), Sara Banks (1996), and Jean-Pierre Lepine (2004) report anywhere from 35 to 54 percent of people who have chronic pain suffer from a diagnosable depression. Those statistics are a little discouraging but verify the close and interacting body-mind correlation between the depression and pain. This relationship suggests that although the depression that accompanies pain is not your fault, there are body-mind practices that can help you to alleviate it. So read on for healing insights and to learn about the reparative yoga practices that are wonderful medicine.

In part, pain and depression are closely linked due to biology. They share some of the same nerve pathways and some of the same chemical messengers, namely serotonin and norepinephrine, that travel between nerves. Both chronic pain and chronic depression can alter how your nervous system functions, which affects how well your mood is moderated. And when your mood is no longer well regulated, pain and sadness intensify. Each heightens the perception of the other in what becomes a self-perpetuating cycle. Joined together, pain and sadness can erode hope, wear you down, and zap your interest in life. The result can be utter misery.

A body-mind experience, depression also shows up in your thoughts. The depressing thoughts that show up when you have pain typically focus on how awful the pain is, how much better it used to be, why this had to happen to you anyway, and how your life is worse off. Such thoughts add fuel to the smoldering flames of depression.

Pain and depression so mutually influence one another that just being depressed puts you at greater risk of experiencing pain. Lepine (2004) found that 80 percent of depressed people receiving outpatient medical care reported painful somatic symptoms. In fact, sometimes depression is primarily experienced as aches and pain and fatigue. Headaches, abdominal distress, and sleep difficulties frequently accompany depression, and because depression is so intertwined with your body, you may not know that you are depressed.

Irritability

Irritability often accompanies depression and can even be its primary expression. When you are irritable you are extremely sensitive to what is going on around you. It is as though your nerves have unraveled and are exposed. Irritability is a state of reactivity that causes you to snap at people and be impatient with them. You feel disagreeable and probably just want to be left alone. Because you are easily annoyed, you might unintentionally push people away and end up without the social support you so need.

Pain and irritability go hand in hand. Pain, especially when it throbs and jolts, causes you to be on edge, unable to be soothed. Pain like that drains your coping skills and leaves you emotionally raw. You are less able to reason clearly or to muster up goodwill. When irritability strikes, you have little to give to yourself and even less to give to others. Probably the best thing to do at that time is to nap, take a shower, stroll outdoors, or do something else that is soothing for you. (By the way, there are several self-soothing lists available online that may give you ideas.)

Anxiety

When you have physical pain, you probably also experience dread and anxiety. When pain is too much or lasts too long, your mind is likely to react with "please, no more" thoughts about pain recurring or worsening over time. "I can't bear more" thoughts escalate pain because they trigger your body's fear response. Also, it is pretty hard to be optimistic when the future looks bleak to your mind.

Optimism, which includes a positive outlook, has a significant impact on your mood and health. So as challenging as it is to muster up optimism, you can learn how to do it by reading the following sections.

First, here is a little information on optimism. V. M. Ferreira and A. M. Sherman (2007) found that optimism partially mediated the relationship of pain to life satisfaction. However, this is not blind or passive optimism. It is an active optimism. In fact, Jill Neimark (2007) found that a hopeful attitude is less important than behavior in determining optimism. This is the encouraging part. Optimism is one part thinking to two parts of doing. It is doing in spite of physical discomfort and mental worry. It is being persistent and taking steps, including making contact with others. The substance of optimism is saying, "Yes, I can," and then doing one thing. Optimism is motion over emotion, taking one step when you feel upset. Optimism alleviates anxiety because it encourages you to act even when you are afraid. In contrast, pessimism is emotion over motion, not taking one step when you feel lousy. Anxiety causes pessimism when it stops action in its tracks and pessimism causes anxiety when it convinces you that you are not capable. For instance, when your mind is under fear's grip, it says, "I can't do this." Then it is your mind, not your physical discomfort, that causes you to recoil from doing what you need or truly want to do.

In all fairness to your body, it is natural that pain causes fear of physical movement. Pain, your body's signal that something is amiss, ushers in thoughts of caution. Realistically, hesitancy may be wise; however, not moving may not be. Avoiding physical movement can have far-reaching consequences. Fear of pain can hold you back from rehabilitative therapies, exercise, and pleasurable outings. Of course, you may have to modify, but better to make adjustments than to be immobilized. The unfortunate consequences of inactivity—increased pain and fatigue, decreased mobility, and fewer social outlets—just reinforce pessimism and fear. This vicious cycle is one that you can interrupt with the practices we teach you later in this chapter.

Additionally, pain may increase the likelihood of having other anxiety symptoms such as flashbacks and nightmares. At least that seems to be the case when injury is related to car accidents and may well be true for injury from other accidents. According to Edward Hickling and Edward Blanchard (2006), 50 percent of people who have been injured in motor-vehicle accidents for which medical care is needed suffer from flashbacks of the accident, frequent nightmares, fear of driving, and extreme anxiety when returning to the site of the accident.

Practices and Meditations for Physical and Emotional Pain

You may not be able to make pain go away, but how you tend to it can make a world of difference in its intensity and in the quality of your life. There is a lot you can do to contribute to your well-being, even if you have to be on pain medications. As Richard Besdine (2011) reported, there are alternative ways to manage chronic pain, including gentle yoga exercises. Said a yoga practitioner who has come through unrelenting trauma and illness, "Yoga is my life-line. My body is distorted and I have to modify poses, but gentle yoga, with its emphasis on breathing and compassion, keeps me going so that I can be there for my kids." There is also a wealth of research, beginning with Jon Kabat Zinn's work at the University of Massachusetts in the 1980s. His major contributions verify the quieting effect of meditation and show that the concentration and observational skills acquired during meditation can effectively reduce chronic pain. There is hope and help.

Dealing with Sleep Deprivation

When it comes to how much you sleep and how deep your sleep is, your lifestyle choices matter. And high on the list of importance, according to yoga, is practicing nonviolence. Yoga sutra 11.35, as interpreted by Mukunda Stiles (2002, 25), reads as follows: "By abiding in nonviolence, one's presence creates an atmosphere in which hostility ceases." Basically, nonviolence is about making wise choices that cultivate a loving, calm atmosphere inside of and around you. These choices include how you interact with others and what you take into your body and mind. Obviously, when you go to bed at night you take the effects of your choices with you.

You are more likely to get a good night's sleep when you feel peaceful inside rather than agitated. For example, even if you are generally a sound sleeper, you can probably recall sleeping poorly one night after having harsh words with a loved one. Having difficult conversations at night when you are exhausted is not the best choice in timing.

A full night's sleep is a lot easier to come by when you have a clean conscience (created by ethical decision making) and an undisturbed mind (created by wise choices about what you look at, listen to, taste, smell, and touch). We repeat: it is all about making wise choices. One important choice is to limit voluntary consumption of violence that revs up your body's fight-or-flight response and fills your mind with images of life as mostly dangerous. Specifically, to improve your sleep, avoid optional exposure to violence on television and in news media, movies, and conversations, especially in the evening hours. Simply stated, do not take violence to bed with you. If you are a trauma survivor, consider this. You did not choose your trauma, but now you have choice about what you put into your mind and body.

To prepare for sleep, be intentional with your sleep hygiene so that you create an inner atmosphere conducive to sleep. Give as much time to purifying your mind as you give to cleansing your body. Here are a few suggestions for creating a nurturing nighttime practice:

- Do something relaxing for your body, such as a couple of gentle stretches (the seated and/or lying-down yoga poses outlined in chapter 4).

- Spend some time snuggling with pets or loved ones.

- Wash the day off of your body with soap and water.

- Take a saltwater bath and visualize impurities and stress flowing down the drain along with the salt (a purifying, cleansing practice recommended by our colleague Ellie Finlay).

- Fill your mind with love and inspiration by listening to a beautiful song, reading scripture, writing in a gratitude journal, meditating, or praying.

Even with good care, sleep can be elusive. During restless nights, when you are uncomfortable, your mind is likely to produce thoughts that distress you. Since you are going to think anyway, be intentional about the contents of your thoughts and turn to your mantra. Sleepless nights are a profound opportunity to recite brief prayers, scriptures, and sacred mantras over and over and over.

Mantras occupy your mind, distract you from pain, and fill you with the energy of love and connection. If you are going to be awake, you may as well be as comfortable as possible. Reciting a mantra has a calming effect. In the beginning of your practice, however, your mind may drift from your mantra to fretting thoughts. When you realize that other thoughts have grabbed your attention, refocus on your mantra and notice your body relax again. You may slip into sleep—and if not, at least you and your mantra are keeping yourself comfortable.

MANTRAS FOR SLEEP

Recite mantras with reverence and respect so that the practice is a body-mind-spirit contemplation rather than a simple concentration exercise. Let yourself feel the emotional-spiritual energy of the words you recite. Fewer words are generally better so that the mantra is simple and focused. Following are types of mantras that you may like to silently recite at night.

- **Self-love mantra:** Recite a vow of love and loyalty to yourself, adapted from the teachings of Thich Nhat Hanh. Select words that you yearn to hear. Examples include "My dear, I am here" and "It's okay; I am here."

- **Present-moment comfort mantra:** Coordinate your words with your breath. For example, whisper "I am here" with the inhalation and "and safe" with the exhalation.

- **Surrender to the divine mantra:** An example is "Thy will."

- **Short scriptural phrase:** An example is "I am with you always."

Focused Attention Meditation for Pain

Samatha, or focused attention meditation, trains you to focus on spiritual qualities. *Samatha*, a Sanskrit word, means "calm abiding." Whether you concentrate on your breath, a mantra, heart energy, or even gazing at a sacred symbol, your single-pointed concentration settles and soothes your mind. This is so helpful when your mind is recoiling from physical and emotional pain.

The first focal-point option is breath, which helps you to access the spiritual quality of stillness. This is perhaps the most researched *samatha* meditation for pain management.

The second focal-point option is the center of your chest, or heart chakra. Heart-focused meditation softens the heartbreak of pain by focusing your attention on the energy of compassion. As sutra 1.36, as interpreted by Stiles (2002, 11), states, "The mind can also find peace by contemplating the luminous light, arising from the heart, which is the source of true serenity." Focusing on your heart causes you to become more aware of its healing energy and may even increase it, as research shows. Antoine Lutz (2008) studied the effect of meditating with the sole focus of generating a state of unconditional loving-kindness and found that focusing on heartfelt compassion activates neural pathways linked to empathy and emotional stability.

The third focal-point option is the silent recitation of a spiritual mantra, which focuses attention on your connection with the sacred. Mantra recitation is an effective way to cope with pain. In fact, Amy Wachholtz and Kenneth Pargament (2005) found that reciting a spiritual mantra (reciting God's name) is more effective than reciting a secular mantra (no religious content) in coping with intense discomfort. In 2008 their additional research found that a regular practice of spiritual mantra recitation is more effective than secular mantra recitation in reducing the severity of migraines in frequent headache sufferers.

The fourth focal-point option is gazing at a sacred object. This option, also known as *gazing concentration meditation*, was discussed in chapter 2. While gazing at a sacred object, symbol, or picture of a spiritual being, look softly and let your eyes blink naturally.

In *samatha* meditation, you focus and refocus. Of course, you cannot refocus until you are aware that your attention has drifted, which means that you are developing two skills: concentration and observation. Maclean (2010) reported that by doing so, you activate areas of the brain responsible for maintaining focus and processing emotions. Amazingly, this not only helps you deal with pain, but changes the nature of pain before it is perceived.

All in all, the research is promising. Take a look at one more study. Fadel Zeidan and colleagues (2011) found that doing concentration meditation using breath awareness in the midst of experiencing pain reduces pain intensity. They found that the somatosensory cortex, the part of the brain that is active during pain, showed little activity during meditation. This suggests that meditation reduces pain by reducing the actual sensation of pain.

Learn this meditation when your pain is lower because it is much easier to learn and concentrate when you are calm. Practice when you are reasonably comfortable. Then, when you need refuge from pain, your practice is there, like a friend, to help you. You might find one practice to be generally soothing and another practice to be more helpful during pain spikes. As a daily practice, Rick found gazing at a sacred object, specifically the beauty of nature, something that inspires a sense of peace and serenity for him, to be very helpful. Focusing on a peaceful scene beyond the pain in his body comforted him. With a cat in his lap, he sat in a chair and looked out at our water garden. During his season of incapacitation, he often stated, "Gazing at the water garden is such a pleasing distraction." However, when he was in agony the best he could do was put his attention right into the middle of the pain and breathe, and breathe some more. "During those times all I could do was surrender to the pain and breathe," Rick recalls. "Spikes of pain at times would take my breath away, but breath always came back, as reliably as a dear friend, available for me to once again focus on it."

INSTRUCTIONS FOR FOCUSED ATTENTION MEDITATION

Experiment for yourself. Choose from the four focal points, ideally one that you find pleasant. Here are a few considerations: If you are new to meditation, it may be easier to focus on a mantra or the movement of breath at your nostrils because they are fixed points of reference. When mental or physical pain is particularly high, a breath focus may be easier to follow than a heart focus because it may be the stronger sensation of the two. Or you may prefer sacred-object focus, since it centers your attention outside of your body. Also, try rocking back and forth slightly. You may find the sensation soothing, or you may prefer utter stillness. Adapt the practice so that you stay in your comfort zone.

Predetermine a time of day and a length of time for your meditation. At first, set a timer to release the need to look at your watch. (Going to the same place at the same time establishes meditation as a habit.) Sit in an upright position to promote alertness unless you need to position your body another way so that you feel at ease. Select a focal point (your breath, your heart chakra, a mantra, or a sacred object) and then attempt to sustain it. When your attention wanders, gently bring it back.

Breathing Practice for Mental and Physical Pain

Learning to breathe deeply and fully is essential for healing. Pain, in the form of sharp physical sensations or surges of fear, can leave you breathless. Breath naturally fluctuates, and breathing shallowly momentarily probably does not harm you, but when pain is chronic, shallow breathing can become chronic as well—and that takes a toll on your health. In brief, here is why: When breath is restricted, exhalations are not full and your lungs are unable to remove stale air and the residual buildup of toxins. Also, when your lungs are not emptied there is less room for the next oxygen-rich inhalation that your body needs in order to be healthy.

Doing an intentional practice resets breathing patterns so that your breath is more optimal. Proper breathing works your lungs, moves your diaphragm, exercises the muscles around your ribs, improves your posture, and supplies an adequate amount of oxygen to your brain and organs. Not only that, it creates pleasant sensations in your body and puts your body at ease. And if you are like most, your body needs many relaxing experiences so that you recognize what being relaxed feels like.

Another benefit of a regular breathing practice is that it develops your capacity to deepen your breath when you need to. That way, when your pain level goes up, you remember to breathe fully into the emotional and physical discomfort. Breathing through painful sensations is an act of compassion because meeting pain with breath softens its edges. Also, when you breathe intentionally, some of your attention shifts away from pain and focuses on breath-

161

ing. This changes your experience from just having pain to having pain and breathing through it.

We really encourage you to incorporate a short breathing practice into your daily routine. It just takes a few minutes and the resolve to do so. Following is a breathing practice that uses deep abdominal breathing as its basis and builds upon it.

DIRGHA PRANAYAMA OR THREE-PART BREATH PRACTICE

This practice gradually deepens your breath. Please do not strain or force. Stay in your "easy does it" zone. Sit comfortably or lie on your back with your eyes closed. Being prone has some advantage because you can noticeably feel the movement of your ribs and torso as breath enters and leaves. Begin by breathing in through your nose for five counts and out for five counts a couple of times to relax your breath.

Next, place your hand on your lower abdomen, below your belly button. Breathe in through your nose and gently expand your belly like you are filling up a balloon. Breathe out and feel your belly contract. Do this breath three to five times. (You may also place a book on your stomach to help increase sensation in the area that is moving in and out.)

Place your hand at the base of your ribs, a couple inches above your belly button. Breathe in and fill your belly, then begin to fill your lower lungs with air. Feel your hand move out as your lungs fill. Then breathe out, first from your lower lungs, then from your belly. Do this cycle three to five times.

Place your hand on your upper chest. Breathe in through your nose and fill your belly, then your lower lungs, and then your upper chest with air so that you feel your heart rise. When you are full of breath, breathe out through your nose, from your upper chest, lower lungs, and finally from your belly. Do this cycle three to five times.

As you practice, focus on your inhalation and exhalation being equal in length. Over time, allow the movement of the breath to be smooth and seamless.

Deep Relaxation

Self-care is crucial when you have mental and physical pain, including taking time for quiet relaxation. Of all the yoga poses, *shavasana*, or final resting pose (see the exercise and illustration for "Final Resting Pose" in chapter 4), is perhaps the most important, especially when pain and upset keep your body and mind agitated. It is important to not skip final resting pose at the end of your yoga practice. It's also healing to practice it by itself another time during the day for ten to thirty minutes.

Shavasana is designed for deep relaxation. It begins with lying down on your back. If possible, lie on the floor, rather than on a bed, to distinguish this from nap time. Let your eyes close. Take a few deep breaths, using three-part breath. Next, scan your body from your toes to your head for muscular tension, and release tension with a few repetitive, gentle shaking motions. Then release efforts to breathe deeply or do anything at all. Simply rest. If your mind gets busy, focus gently on your body or breath. When your mind becomes quiet again, simply rest.

Sadly, many people do not know how to relax; for people who are driven or restless this pose is not easy. So if you are not inclined to take rest, experiment with lying down for just a few minutes. Let yourself acclimate to the experience. The benefits are well worth the effort, because taking frequent rest breaks teaches you how pleasurable being relaxed truly is. It also calms your mind, unwinds tension, and allows your body to heal.

Healing Painful Emotions with Breath, Understanding, and Focus

How trauma affects you depends in large part upon how you care for the emotional pain that follows. Grief is natural and, when accepted, heals you. Other emotions associated with trauma—such as sadness, fear, and anger—when not taken care of can linger and further wound you. However, when cared for they become a rich part of human living that helps you to understand yourself.

Here are two fundamental points to remember in learning to take care of your emotions: First, you are more than your emotions, no matter how awful they feel. Who you are cannot be reduced to changeable emotions. It is simply part of your human nature to experience emotions. However moved you are by them, they are like waves that rise and fall in the ocean. The ocean is not defined by its waves any more than you are defined by emotions.

Second, breath is your greatest emotional regulator. Intentionally breathing through emotional pain helps you to not totally collapse into it. This is especially important when painful emotions become chronic. Breath focus steadies you so that you are not totally submersed. It takes some practice to not be swept under, but you are not doomed to a life of just one painful emotion. You can have a full range of emotions that include hope, courage, and contentment.

Let us begin with grief, that painful emotion that comes in the aftermath of loss. Grief can be very encompassing for some time when loss is great. Yet it lessens. With deep compassion for yourself, breathe into the grief, allow it, and feel it pass through. Powerful waves of grief may take your breath away, but waves do subside, giving you a chance to breathe fully before the next wave arrives.

Allowing grief deepens your understanding of life's seasons and connects you with others. For example, Mary's younger sister tragically died thirty years ago, and we recently attended a graveside service next to the plot where her sister's body was buried. When Mary walked by Bev's gravestone she burst into tears. Once again, like an ocean swell, raw grief swept through her—and then subsided. As evidence of its healing properties, grief left Mary feeling tender, prompting her to warmly embrace others attending the funeral whom she may otherwise have had more superficial contact with.

Some emotions move through you and cause you to feel freer, similar to the way grief opened Mary's heart at the funeral. Other times, emotions become long lasting and keep trauma alive, until you understand them and learn how to take care of yourself when they arise. Another example comes from Betty, a woman with a big heart. She experienced years of sadness after getting out of an oppressive marriage. She often cried and felt hopeless, convinced that she was permanently messed up. Crying did not provide relief, offer insight, or move her toward renewed intimacy with life. Even breathing through her tears, while helpful, was not healing enough. She felt discouraged and needed to find a way to feel encouraged. One day it dawned on her that she ached to be emotionally supported and she vowed to begin encouraging herself.

Betty learned to shift her focus from discouraging thoughts and emotions to words that encourage her. Now when she feels down she says, "You're okay; I am here. Let's get up and do something." She moves into action, even if it is just washing dishes. Then she goes on to another task, such as going to the grocery store. Then she moves to something else, such as calling her sister. All the while, if she has to, she whispers, "You're okay; I am here." For her, focusing on encouraging words is a challenging but beneficial practice that pulls her out of old emotional pain and into her current life.

Learning to focus and to be selective about what you focus on is central to the practice of yoga. In fact, according to T. K. V. Desikachar (1995), sutra 2.29 states that *dharana*, or the ability to direct your mind, is a fundamental component of yoga. Focusing is also central in dealing with chronic emotional pain. You do not have to be at the mercy of old pain. You can direct your mind to thoughts that encourage and uplift you.

FOCUS ON IDEAS AND IMAGES THAT FILL YOU WITH LIFE-ENHANCING EMOTIONS

This practice is for you if you are prone to discouragement, exhaustion, feeling overwhelmed, or other persistent, painful emotions. This practice is for you if you need to feel courage, relief, strength, peace, or hope. First, determine which emotion you want to feel. Then come up with a memory, story, song, poem, image, or phrase that you associate with the healing emotion or energy you desire. Search until you find the right words, song, or image.

Following are some ideas to prompt your inquiry.

- **Words spoken or songs sung by a loving relative.** For example, if you need strength and your aunt hummed her way through great difficulties, call upon her for help. In your memory of her is the strength you need. See her in your mind's eye and hum like she hummed.

- **Scriptural text or spiritual saying.** For example, if you need courage and know a scriptural story that evokes courage, whisper it when you feel frightened.

- **Spiritual song or childhood lullaby.** For example, if you need peace and know a song that evokes peace, sing that when you feel agitated.

- **Quote from a hero or heroine.** For example, if you need perseverance, think of a movie or book character who remained true to his or her values and followed his or her dreams even when times were tough. Call upon his or her words when you want to give up.

- **Healing words written on at least three sticky notes.** Frame the notes and post them where you will see them several times daily so that you do not forget.

Remember, this is a skill that takes some practice to cultivate. Focus on your breath and speak or sing your words daily. Then you are able to focus on healing words when painful emotions arise.

Surrender to the Divine

Perhaps the most powerful way to deal with emotional and physical pain is a daily spiritual practice that includes giving your pain over to a higher power. More than just handing over pain, spiritual practice is about an intimate relationship with the divine. Yoga sutra 1.22, as translated by Stiles (2002, 7), states, "The end of spiritual practice is only attained by placing oneself in the Lord."

Sadhana, a Sanskrit word, refers to a discipline that is a means of accomplishing something. A spiritual discipline is turning again and again to a relationship with the sacred. Rick's mother's practice was an early-morning soak in a small indoor pool. Shortly after waking up she slipped her pain-ridden body into the still, quiet warm water, where she remained for an hour. She hummed songs, talked with God, and enjoyed being weightless and pain-free. Alone in her water sanctuary she occasionally wept. Then she rose up out of the water, dried herself off, and went about her day. Faithfully, morning after morning, she submersed herself into her water ritual.

Pain often intensifies spiritual yearning. Severe and chronic pain can drop you to your knees in a cry for mercy. If you ache to receive spiritual sustenance, it is there for the asking. As Stiles's (2002) interpretation of sutra 1.21 states, "For those who have an intense urge for Spirit and wisdom, it sits near them, waiting." This sutra suggests that great desire, not belief, draws you to spirit.

Summary

Many people experience trauma and pain. Although pain is deeply personal, it is shared by many. Physical pain, when it is intense and/or chronic, is associated with loss, grief, sleep disturbance, and emotional pain that, when not lovingly tended to, can be long lasting. Fortunately you do not have to remain stuck in painful states. Research shows that yogic practices of breathing, concentration on life-affirming emotions, nonviolence, mantra recitation, deep relaxation, spiritual discipline, and surrender to the divine help you to accept, modulate, and reduce pain. They also teach you to take care of yourself in the midst of pain by focusing on emotional energies that heal, turning to comforting words for strength and relying on the sacred for strength and peace.

chapter 7

trauma, difficult life transitions, and the spiritual journey

trauma and difficult life transitions are often intertwined. The aftermath of trauma can bring about difficulties in adjusting to life changes, such as what a veteran might experience when reintegrating back into civilian life after coming home from a war zone. Likewise, difficult life transitions, such as a midlife divorce, can bring up memories of betrayal, abuse, and lack of nurturance in earlier life. During times of trauma and transition, your relationship with the sacred often comes to the forefront. Both can send you on a search for spiritual sustenance that may result with the sacred taking up more space in your life.

To address these topics, we start with a discussion on trauma and difficult transitions, as well as the significance of spirituality in coping and healing. Then we explore three ways of experiencing the sacred—spiritual coping, loss of the spiritual connection, and spiritual transformation, as identified by Kenneth Pargament (2007)—as they pertain to healing from trauma. Last, we turn to the teachings of the yoga sutras of Patanjali for guidance along the spiritual journey.

Trauma, Difficult Transitions, and Healing

As we have previously stated, in varying degrees, emotional trauma fractures trust, wounds human dignity, and shatters faith. And sometimes the effect is great. As David Elkins (1995, 91) wrote, "Some violations and betrayals ... wound so deeply that they can only be called abuses to the soul." Those kinds of traumas reverberate through all domains of life, including how secure you feel in your own skin and who you feel safe with. It is no wonder then that trauma can lead to significant changes in your relationships with family, friends, and work.

How does emotional trauma affect transition? Rich Morin (2011) reports that a Pew Research Center survey on military veterans found that emotional trauma is associated with a more difficult transition back to civilian life than physical injury. Also, military personnel are more likely to experience emotional trauma than physical injury. This survey found that 43 percent of veterans who served in the last decade reported a military-related experience that they found to be "emotionally traumatic or distressing," and 16 percent suffered a serious physical injury. Clearly, acute and chronic exposure to violence, hatred, bullying, and threat of injury can take a tremendous toll.

Major life changes—especially when associated with loss, injury, and trauma—thrust you, sooner or later, into the realms of meaning, purpose, and spirituality. Potentially life-altering, these times are unforgettably imprinted into your life, not just because they change outer circumstances but because they are doors to your soul that reveal the deeper dimensions of life. When this happens you no longer perceive life or experience life in the same way.

Transitions change who you are, as you grow or decay but do not remain the same. Undesired transitions such as those associated with divorce, death of a loved one, and traumatic incidences initially feel decompensating. When this occurs, your coping skills no longer keep you and your life functioning as usual. Certain aspects of your life that you had put together fall apart. Before moving forward you are thrust back into the inner world of uncertainty and unresolved trauma from the past, including childhood, no matter how many years ago that was.

This in-between period is a crucial time. The life that was is gone, leaving you, at least for some time, with an unclear picture of where life is taking you. In transition, you have some healing to do. This is an invitation to go into the world of psyche; however, doing so may not be easy. Entering into inner life is a catalyst to healing, when done wisely and with support. The other option, not looking within, may result in a collapse into addictions, sustained

171

emotional distress, and/or a deteriorating lifestyle. If you go there for a while, let it just be a while. You do not have to remain stuck.

Since adverse transitions can result in decline or growth, it is important to look at what healing entails. Although there is no set formula for healing, there are markers along the way. This is true for traumas that are recent and for those that happened many years ago. Even if trauma has held you back for many years, you can still engage in a healing journey.

Knowing about the milestones of healing helps you to identify where you are in the recovery process. After an acute trauma, there is an initial period of shock and turbulence. It takes a good amount of time to recognize the extent of damage. This is particularly true when dealing with trauma of emotional maltreatment because it is often hidden from the public and denied or minimized. Then, as healing progresses, it does not move in a linear direction. Like a spiral, it circles around, inching closer to your heart and to the truth as it progresses. Along the way, you pass through the following milestones as many times as it takes for healing to touch the deepest recesses of your being. The five milestones are:

1. Accepting the reality of what happened and what is changed,

2. Gradually letting go of the past,

3. Having optimism for the future,

4. Living with meaning and fulfillment in the present, and

5. Experiencing an abiding sense of self-worth.

If life is still marred by the past there is hope. You can continue to heal. Healing is truly the journey of a lifetime, and, as you are about to read, turning to the sacred is the ultimate source of sustenance along the way.

Even research verifies the healing power of the divine, as the following studies on war and sexual trauma demonstrate. Morin

(2011) found that religious faith, measured by how often a recent veteran attends religious services, is one of the more significant factors in having an easy reentry. Gregory Knapik and his colleagues (2010) found that connecting to others in spiritual settings and connecting with a divine being or higher power are helpful in coping with sexual violence. Earlier studies (Glaister and Able 2001; Smith and Kelly 2001) also found that belief in and connection with a higher power aids recovery from sexual violence. Annick Shaw and colleagues (2005) indicated that spirituality is beneficial to the healing of trauma victims. If you have suffered from what seems unspeakable, let this body of evidence nudge you toward the spiritual.

You do not even have to define yourself as religious to move toward the sacred. If you are spiritual but not religious, you have a lot of company. There are resources in the following sections that are suitable for believers and nonbelievers.

For the sake of clarity, *spirituality* pertains to your relationship with an ultimate reality or higher power. *Religiousness*, in contrast, refers to religious activity, such as church attendance and dedication to and belief in a religious doctrine. Spirituality may or may not occur within the context of religious life. Daniel Stone (2009) reported on a *Newsweek* survey that found nearly half of the Americans surveyed described themselves as both religious and spiritual while 30 percent said they were spiritual but not religious. However you define ultimate reality or higher power, the spiritual journey is a personal, intimate path of discovering the sacred nature of all life, including your own. Spiritual practices, including meditation, prayer, and contemplation, are intended to develop your sense of connectedness with the larger reality of the divine.

Spirituality as a Resource for Coping

Suffering causes a search for meaning and comfort. During darkest times you are likely to turn to religion or spirituality to connect with the sacred, whether or not you come from a strong faith background. For instance, most people turned toward the sacred for support after September 11, 2001. According to Mark Schuster and colleagues (2001), more than 80 percent of people in a random sample across the United States said that they coped with their feelings after the disaster by turning to religion. Therefore it is not surprising that religion is the most frequently turned to resource for dealing with trauma and difficult transitions.

We can turn to Mary for a personal example of turning to religion as a way of coping. After a younger sister and her father unexpectedly died in 1982, Mary and the rest of her family were devastated. Five months later, Mary and her husband moved from Iowa to Oklahoma. Bereaved, away from family and friends, and reeling from uprising memories of incest, she began attending a church that felt compatible with her agnostic bent. For the first time since graduating from high school, Mary turned toward the sacred, as unsure as she was about what that was. Sunday after Sunday she sat in a pew and sobbed, grieving her sister's death and a whole lot more. The sun-filled sanctuary, the music, and the message from the pulpit soothed her broken heart.

When feeling broken and alone you ache for relationship with something that comprehends the incomprehensible and comforts that which can't be comforted, which is why people are apt to turn toward the divine. There are many ways to seek intimacy with ultimate reality. Whether through prayer, reciting God's name, solitude, religious services, meditation, or time in nature, your effort expresses, in the words of Thomas Merton (1969, 82), a "yearning for the simple presence of God." Like many others, when feeling stressed and isolated, Mary sought out the divine because she did not know what else to turn to. According to Pargament (2007), turning to the divine is especially helpful if you are experiencing a hardship and have few personal and social resources, as was the case for Mary. On the other hand, if you have an established spiritual life you are likely to seek solace in your personal practices, and if you are a member of a religious community you typically draw comfort from shared rituals.

Even if you currently define yourself as nonreligious, during painful times you may seek a personal relationship with a higher power. Mary, who had turned away from organized religion and spirituality during college, found a way to reconnect. "As a young teenager I loved to sit on the end of a pew close to my favorite stained-glass window during church services," she recalls. "There, bathed in the light shining through the window, I felt loved, safe, and understood. Although unable to connect with the doctrine being taught, the rays of sunlight that touched me felt holy. Years later, sitting in that sunny sanctuary in Tulsa, I felt that same presence."

Whether it's sitting by a church window or listening to the sound of a beautiful bell, sacred rituals—including ceremonies, songs, and prayers—are filled with energy and potential. And sacred objects such as cathedrals, sculptures, and rosaries, far from inert, are "vital objects" (LaMothe 1998). Sacred rituals and objects are spiritual resources that infuse you with the divine. They are not short-term problem-solving devices, although they do give ways to approach and contextualize difficulties. Spiritual resources have the capacity to soothe and comfort, inspire and empower (Greenberg et al. 1995). Fundamentally, spiritual resources facilitate your spiritual journey, helping you to access the energy of compassion, unity, surrender, hope, forgiveness, and understanding. Along the way, they give spiritual meaning to traumatic events. This may take some time, but when understood through a spiritual perspective, painful, even violent experiences are placed in a more benevolent context: one that offers hope (Park 2005).

Loss of Spiritual Connection

It may be that turning to the sacred does not comfort, seem desirable, or even possible, at least for some period of time. For

175

instance, you may have felt wounded by the doctrine or the leaders of your childhood church. For obvious reasons, religious abuse can turn you away from the sacred. Additionally, other childhood traumas, such as sexual abuse and other forms of violence, can turn you off to the divine. Once again, research shows this to be the case. Kane, Cheston, and Greer (1993) reported that those sexually abused as a child may view God in a negative light. Alex Bierman (2005) also found a negative relationship between childhood mal-treatment and religiousness, particularly when abuse was by fathers. This makes sense, because if your father was harsh and unpredict-able, you may have formed a negative view of father figures, and in some religions a higher power is depicted in paternal imagery.

Transition, when coupled with the uprising of old trauma, can put emotional and spiritual life in great upheaval. Let's say, for instance, that after your long-term spouse commits suicide you discover that your partner had lived a double life. Things were not as they seemed. You were deceived and betrayed. Not surprising, you feel a multitude of emotions, including feeling abandoned. However, if you were emotionally malnourished as a child, all these years later, you may also feel abandoned by childhood caretakers and by the divine and lose interest in the spiritual life.

Likewise, a major crisis with your teenage son can trigger old emotions. When your child is in an ongoing state of need or trouble, the kind that can have devastating consequences, anger, distress, or grief from your childhood may be activated. You may also question if there really is a God or why God allows terrible things to happen. Exhausted and discouraged, you may give up on the divine.

Even when trauma shakes your spiritual life the spark is prob-ably not fully snuffed out. It may smolder under ashes of disappoint-ment and pain and then be rekindled. You may yearn to turn to its light and warmth at another time, including when you experience another trauma, feel terribly, alone and/or see life being ruined by an addiction.

Spiritual Transformation

One way or another, sooner or later, you may begin centering your life on the sacred. Often, the process begins with attending church services, praying for relief and comfort, walking in solitude, taking yoga classes, learning to meditate, or hearing an inspirational speaker; then it progresses over time. You may feel an inexplicable sense of not being alone at times, such as during prayerful silence, watching the sun rise, or resting in a yoga pose. On the other hand, you may have some experience that rapidly draws you into relationship with the sacred. However slowly or quickly spiritual life evolves, it includes calling upon the divine for guidance, spending time in spiritual practices, and contextualizing life through the lens of the divine.

As a relationship with the sacred becomes real and deep, you feel stronger and have more insights into your life. This enables you to gently approach trauma with compassion and understanding. Gradually, you feel less shattered by the past, worry less about the future, and turn to spiritual practices for sustenance. Feeling connected with the sacred, you feel more peaceful and life seems friendlier.

Even if maltreatment causes you to be less religious, at some point you may turn toward spirituality as a resource for healing. Look at what research found. Patricia Ryan (1998) indicated that while some victims of abuse turn away from religion, many consider their abusive experiences to be catalysts for an increased sense of spirituality. Sannisha Dale and Jessica Daniel (2011) conducted a literature review that revealed that while some survivors of childhood violence denounce religion altogether, many alter their spiritual practices, change faith, or turn to a more personal form of spiritual practice. Undeniably, you are in the company of many people who have suffered and found their way to a closer relationship with the sacred.

Sometimes the divine touch is dramatic, especially when it comes in the form of spiritual experiences. Impossible to fully describe, spiritual experiences are events filled with wonder, awe, reverence, humility, and surrender before the experience of something great. Life altering, they help you give up addictions, understand trauma experiences from a spiritual perspective, and have greater faith.

One way to appreciate the power of spiritual experiences is to look to the life of saints, many of whom suffered great trauma. For instance, St. Francis of Assisi's powerful spiritual experiences motivated him to leave behind his military career and begin a new life. A revered saint, his love of animals and beautiful prayers live on. Rabia, an Islamic saint, spent many years in a life of slavery, abuse, and forced prostitution. Her mystical experiences of God motivated a patron to buy her freedom. She became a beloved saint who healed many and whose poetry transmits the highest compassion.

The spiritual journey can take other paths, as was the experience of Mother Teresa, who often felt spiritually alone. She felt pain and darkness in her soul yet radiated the light of the divine. In her letters, collected by Brian Kolodiejchuk (2007), she writes about the anguish of not feeling Christ's presence. She spread joy even when she did not feel it and remained close to Jesus in pure faith. Remarkably and powerfully, Mother Teresa was able to transmit compassion to others and eventually find profound peace. We include her story here because if you are in a period of interior emptiness, you may find great comfort in her compelling example.

If you are at all so inclined, do turn to the sacred and to spiritual practices, even if your motivation is that you feel lost and do not know what else to do. At the very least, meditation, prayer, gentle yoga, and practices of compassion quiet the mind and soothe the body. You are going to profit from your efforts and most likely reap tremendous rewards.

Whatever your motivation, we encourage going to meditation or prayer time regularly. In fact, virtually every religious tradition

178

espouses the importance of perseverance in whatever pathway you follow. You do not have to be an expert—simply begin where you are. In fact, you can only start where you are! The practice deepens and benefits become richer over time. Consider this: it took Michelangelo more than four years to paint the ceiling of the Sistine Chapel. As a sculptor, not a painter, he had to learn the medium as he went. Faithfully, day after day, he climbed up the scaffolding, learning as he progressed.

Clearly, it is important to do practices that align with your religious or philosophical orientation. Secular or sacred, meditation practices lead to greater happiness and health. If you do not resonate with the concept of God, yet yearn to have a quiet mind, consider a form of meditation that focuses on inner illumination. Within this context, meditation offers a way to go beneath the outer realms of thoughts and emotions into deeper realms of stillness and consciousness.

One meditation that focuses on inner illumination is *transcendental meditation*, which uses the silent repetition of a word or symbol as its focus. The simple sound moves attention beneath thought into a quiet state of awareness, known as *transcendental consciousness*. In this state of restful alertness, your body gains deep rest and you feel wonderfully peaceful. Joshua Rosenthal and collaborators (2011) found that this meditation, when practiced twice a day for fifteen to twenty minutes, helps relieve symptoms of posttraumatic stress disorder among combat veterans, in part because of the profound healing effect it has on the nervous system.

As James, a war veteran, said, "After coming back from Iraq, I didn't feel and I didn't care. Nothing comforted me, including talking to the chaplain, because I don't believe in the supernatural." After a suicide attempt, he knew he had to do something, so he followed a friend's recommendation to learn meditation. The relief he felt after a few weeks of practicing has motivated him to remain faithful to twice-daily sessions. Committed to a practice compatible with his life philosophy, for the first time in a long time he feels peaceful deep inside.

Yoga and Transformation

In this section we look into a few of the poga sutras of Patanjali for support along your way. In doing so we come to the primary purpose of yoga, which is to know and express your spiritual nature. The *Yoga Sutras of Patanjali*, although not a religious text, is a remarkable treatise that helps you to heal and live out full human potential as a spiritual being. The sutras clearly affirm that you are not the contents of thoughts, that tremendous support is available, and that you are a conscious being capable of great love and wisdom. Transformation does not involve creating a better you, it entails discovering the sacred within and cultivating capacities to be life-loving, intentional, and thoughtful.

Dedication and Persistence

Yoga practices are powerful. However, you have to actually sit on a meditation/prayer cushion or lie on a yoga mat—not just once, but again and again and again, in order to truly transform your life. On the other hand, every practice matters and is a movement into health, peace, and connection.

Gandhi is often quoted as saying, "Be the change you want to see," which implies taking action—daily—to actually experience what you desire. Think about what motivates you to practice yoga or meditation. You might consider the change(s) you want to see and also how the practice affects you. Having some clarity about why you practice makes it easier to be consistent. It is also possible to feel drawn to yoga or meditation without really understanding your motivation. If that is true for you, trust your intuition and the practice.

A yoga friend with a history of childhood and adult family trauma is clear about why she attends four yoga classes weekly. "Having struggled with severe, chronic anxiety in the past, yoga is the medication that keeps me in remission. By slowing down and focusing on breath I am able to tap into my God space, that reservoir of peace that resides deep inside. When I do, the dis-ease of anxiety melts away. Plus, I thoroughly enjoy the practice, which makes it easy to do." Loyal to a yoga practice for more than six years, she credits it with keeping her off of anxiety medications. Our friend knows that wishing to be calm does not produce inner peace, but doing regular yoga practices does.

The sutras stress the importance of an ongoing practice. Mukunda Stiles (2002, 5) interprets sutra 1.14 as saying "that practice is indeed firmly grounded within you when you pursue it incessantly, with reverence, for a long time." Having a practice that you are attracted to makes it easier to stay with it over the long haul, and recognizing that saints and sages have done these practices for centuries helps you to approach practice with reverence. So, begin where you are and let the practice develop over time. If sitting for twenty minutes of meditation is uncomfortable, begin with five or ten minutes and build up over time. Approach practice as a student who is willing to learn. Take classes, talk with a teacher, and/or read books to maximize the benefits of yoga and meditation sessions. Also, be encouraged by the science. The research presented in this book irrefutably states that there is much to gain through regular practice.

We know that it is easy to practice consistently when your mood is up or when you feel desperate and do not know what else to do. Let the spiritual practices done during times of joy and pain intensify your resolve to practice faithfully, no matter what. Simply go to your practice. Practice because you yearn to connect with your deepest inner self. Practice because you know the relief of feeling peaceful. Practice because you do not know where else to turn for comfort. Practice because you have learned to breathe through self-defeating thoughts such as "I don't want to," "It doesn't help," "I can't," or "I hurt too much" and are no longer derailed by them.

James, the war veteran, was clear about his motivation for taking up meditation. He wanted to be comforted and he wanted to live. Although meditating on a mantra was not easy at first, he knew that he had to do something in order to heal, or the effects of war trauma might take his life. He attended classes to learn how to meditate, put a comfortable chair in his bedroom, and sat for fifteen to twenty minutes morning and night. He selected 6:00 a.m. and 6:00 p.m. as his practice time. Having a consistent time helped to establish the habit of regular practice. He told family and friends that he was unavailable during those times and he turned his cell phone off. He felt happier as the months went by, eventually gave up beer drinking, and took up gardening. Now, after a few years of practicing, he says, "I still sit for meditation before breakfast and dinner. I don't miss many days because I don't feel right when I skip. I've grown fond of meditation and that quiet feeling I get. Life isn't perfect; however, I feel a lot more contented and I want to keep it that way."

YOUR PERSONAL
YOGA/MEDITATION PRACTICE

Be intentional. Plan out your practice. Begin with a personally selected practice that interests you. You may choose to attend yoga or meditation classes. You may design a simple home practice that includes gentle stretches, mantra recitation, a breathing practice, and seated meditation. Keep it pleasing so that you want to do your practice. For a home practice, carve out sacred space. Arrange a chair, cushion, or mat in a clean, airy space. Predetermine a practice schedule, including start and stop times. Practice at the same time to help make it a daily habit.

Asking for Support

You are not alone; wise companions are as close as your memory. All you have to do is bring to mind extraordinary people and call upon them to be with you. Thoughts contain energy and earnest thoughts about extraordinary people connect you with the energy they exemplified. Simply spend time with them in prayer, study, and contemplation. According to B. K. S. Iyengar (1993), yoga sutra 1.37 states that you gain inner stability by contemplating on great sages. Daily reflection on beloved spiritual beings develops such intimacy between the two of you that you feel the divinity the other emanates. For example, contemplating the serene state of Buddha causes you to experience serenity. Contemplating the great compassion of Jesus fills you with compassion. In commenting on the same sutra, T. K. V. Desikachar (1995) states that when you have difficulties, seeking the counsel of someone, dead or alive, who has overcome similar problems can be very helpful. So when you go through rough times, do not suffer alone. Ask for help from those who radiate the strength, compassion, or wisdom that you need.

Throughout history there have been many highly evolved individuals. Once again, we offer St. Francis of Assisi as an example. Eknath Easwaran (1994) wrote that by meditating daily on the words of St. Francis, you may find yourself gradually becoming more like him, bringing a little more peace, hope, and love into the world. If his beautiful prayer "Lord, make me an instrument of your peace" touches your heart, do as Mother Teresa did and include St. Francis in your support system. Perhaps recite his prayer before you meditate. Then, call upon his words when you feel injured or despairing. In the moment of reading his prayer you make contact with peace. On rough days fill yourself with the energy of the prayer by reading it morning, noon, and night.

Let your inner support system be large. Include those who made a positive difference in your life. For instance, if your grandmother was a woman of great patience, call on her to help you when you feel impatient. Say, "Grandma, thank you for being patient with me. Be with me now. I need your help." Feel her patience and know that her patience is alive within you. If your schoolteacher believed in you, call upon her when you doubt your own abilities. Say, "Teacher, thank you for believing in me. Be with me now. I need your help." Feel her support and know that her confidence is alive within you.

Widen your internal support group to include animals. In our circle of wise beings is our beloved pet dog, Bubba, who loved scampering in the woods. When he became blind he continued to chase sounds and scents into the woods, even though he inevitably crashed headlong into tree trunks. Limitations did not dampen his enthusiasm. Now, when pain makes life seem too hard, we remember Bubba and say, "Bubba, thank you for your love of life. Be with us now." Next thing we know, we are laughing while we recall a Bubba story. Bubba, and his zest for life, lives on in us.

WRITE ABOUT YOUR INTERNAL SUPPORT SYSTEM

List your primary spiritual teachers. Consider how you contact them. Compile a list of favorite prayers, songs, and scriptures that draws them to you. Next, list people who have significantly contributed to your life, beginning with those you knew as a child, continuing on with those who did or do impact you as an adult. These are people who believe in you, see your potential, stay with you, tell you the truth, and model courage and kindness. Compose a few stories about their influence on you. List animals that modeled unconditional love, forgiveness, fidelity, and ease with life. Write a few heart-melting stories about what they taught you.

Cultivating Life-Affirming Attitudes

The mind is a malleable instrument, one you can develop to be a source of well-being. Amazingly, you do not have to remain trapped in pain-producing thoughts. The more you study your mind and its thoughts, the more you realize how extremely damaging negative thoughts are. Now, if you have been severely mistreated, you may find it difficult to accept the reality that your own thoughts now contribute to your suffering. And yet, that may be the case.

Here is the good news. Here is the truth. You can train yourself to shift attention from misery to well-being. Certainly, doing so is a practice and due to lack of training, most people, ourselves included, fall under the spell of habitual thoughts. However, every intentional life-affirming thought gives immediate benefit and further trains your mind to be an instrument of hope. Plus, cultivating attitudes of love, hope, and contentment sure beats perpetuating attitudes of discontent, fear, despair, and outrage.

The yoga sutras show you how to transform your mind. In this section we turn to yoga sutra 1.33. According to Stiles (2002, 10), this sutra says that "by cultivating attitudes of friendliness towards happiness, compassion toward suffering, delight toward virtue and equanimity toward vice, thoughts become purified and obstacles to self-knowledge are lessened." Promote these attitudes and transform your mind from being an instrument that causes suffering to one that brings happiness to yourself and to others.

Friendliness Toward Happiness

First we look at being friendly toward happiness. Being friendly consists of attitudes and behaviors that welcome, socialize, and approach. Friendliness toward happiness involves noticing it in others and smiling in response. It also includes commenting on your own happy mood when you are happy. Simply saying, "In this moment I am happy" reinforces happiness. If you have suffered from painful moods you may overlook contentment when it arises in you. Remember, what you give attention to grows, so pay attention to moments of happiness. One woman, whose medical maltreatment caused bankruptcy and temporary paralysis, said, "Yoga taught me to choose joy. I conclude my morning prayers by saying, 'Today, I choose joy,' and then I look for joy in the dog's play, the children's laughter, the ability to breathe without a ventilator. I also practice giving big, beaming smiles to others and then take delight in their response. I have found that joy is contagious."

Compassion Toward Suffering

At times suffering is so overwhelming that happiness seems elusive. This is the time to practice compassion. Begin with recognizing whatever emotion you feel. Say, "I feel unhappy" as a way to acknowledge pain, but do not leave yourself alone with dark moods. Reach out with kindness to console yourself. Hug and reassure yourself, write a letter of compassion, recite *Metta* Prayer, put your hand on your heart and breathe. (To review practices of compassion, including *Metta* Prayer, refer back to chapter 1). Focus more on the act of consoling than on the emotion of feeling inconsolable. Pardon mistakes made and be merciful. Say over and over, "It's okay; I forgive you and I will not leave you." Become an instrument of peace. Do this because you are more than the painful emotions that you feel. Do this because, deep inside, you have vast reservoirs of love and understanding. And if you do not believe in your own kind nature, just remember one incident when your heart was touched by the suffering of an animal or child or a loved one. Even remembering the situation probably stirs your heart and, if it does, that is the proof of your loving heart.

Delight in Virtue

Some traumas can feel as though you have been injected with the poison of moral deficiency. In a way you have been, because no one in his or her right mind intentionally harms another. Those who maliciously wound someone else feel disconnected from their own goodness. They do not know that human life is sacred, including their own, probably because they were treated with horrible disrespect when they were young or they have a serious mental illness. Yet the toxins of hatred, revenge, and blaming can be transmitted unto you. When they are, you risk becoming an instrument of destruction, in your own life and in the lives of others.

To cleanse your mind of such poisons, give it big doses of virtue. In addition to cultivating happiness and compassion, take delight in virtue. Celebrating your own and others' virtuous behaviors neutralizes venom in your mind and fills you up with moral excellence. And as you are about to see, taking delight in virtue is easy to do because virtue occurs all around you. You just have to recognize, practice, and celebrate small and large acts of virtue.

First of all, it helps to identify the moral qualities of virtue. They include charity, temperance, chastity, diligence, patience, kindness, and humility. Obvious examples of virtue include pausing to let a motorist into a lane of traffic, crediting those who contributed to success, being sexually faithful to a partner, not giving up when the going is hard, and putting careful thought and research into important decisions.

Virtue is not a heavy burden but an opportunity to express reverence for life. The idea here is to not only practice virtue but to enjoy it wherever and whenever you see it. Celebrating virtue has a redemptive benefit, showing you that human goodness and decency are real and enduring.

Equanimity Toward Vice

Trauma can cause painful reactions of a sense of powerlessness and/or righteousness. If you or a loved one has been horribly mistreated, you may become vindictive, judgmental, or terrified when faced with other injustices. You may even justify cruelty and unintentionally perpetuate the cycle of violence, at least in your thinking if not in your actions.

Equanimity means remaining calm and level-headed when confronted with inequity so that you can make wise choices. You could say that it is the opposite of freaking out! It is also taking care of your upset emotions so that you can reason your way through difficulties.

Practicing equanimity is not about condoning or not reacting to wrongdoing. And as we wrote earlier, equanimity is not about suppressing your emotional responses. After all, you feel whatever emotions you feel. Thinking that you should feel calm does not ease emotional distress. You can practice equanimity when you are upset. It may mean breathing through agitation, talking to yourself in a firm, calm voice when you are overwrought, and giving yourself some time before you respond. It may involve talking things over with others, doing some research, and looking deeply into challenging situations before responding.

The time to practice equanimity is when you feel defensive, build a mental case against someone, feel hatred, or feel too terrified to do what you know you need to do. The ability to remain calm in disturbing circumstances is a mental muscle that is strengthened with practice.

Here is an example. Many years ago we attended a retreat and witnessed a man named Ben lovingly confront the esteemed teacher. A longtime student of the teacher, Ben had been shamed by the teacher in a previous incident. After being humiliated in front of the group, Ben wanted to retaliate. To have some time, he took the afternoon off to journal, meditate, and walk by the lake. He returned to the evening meeting but did not interact because he was still too upset. The following morning Ben was ready. He had written a letter and was prepared to speak. When speaking, he felt very emotional but took care of himself. He breathed deeply when sobbing, paused to calm himself, and continued reading his letter. Speaking his truth directly, yet respectfully, he powerfully modeled equanimity to those of us who were present.

Surrender to the Divine

Surrender is so central to healing that we discussed it in chapter 6 as a way to deal with pain. Surrender is also fundamental to yoga and to centering your life on the sacred. Therefore we discuss it further. First of all, if you are a trauma survivor, please recognize that you cannot endure cruelty and suffering alone, as much as you may try to carry it without help. You need support, not only from others, but also from a loving relationship with higher intelligence. And while surrender may begin by falling on your knees and crying out for help, it does not end there.

Surrender involves bowing down in reverence. Sutra 1.23, as translated by Iyengar (1993, 73), says "that citta [your state of mind] may be restrained by profound meditation upon God and total surrender to Him." In other words, you can feel incredible stillness by deep submission to God. This is a yielding of everything: all virtuous actions, pains, pleasures, joys, and sorrows. Symbolically and perhaps literally, this is an act of prostration, laying down your life to the divine. When you surrender everything at the feet of the divine there is no reason for your mind to be agitated or troubled for there is nothing left for it to do. In the moment of surrender, you give up your worries, plans, disappointments, accomplishments, and expectations. In total renunciation your mind becomes utterly quiet and peaceful.

Surrender can be practiced by offering regular prayers of submission. One retreatant, a woman who courageously divorced her abusive husband, now concludes her evening meditation with this prayer: "I release my sorrow and my joy to you, dear God, and rest in your care." This ritual of submission, which she loves, is deeply embedded because she practices it daily.

Another aspect of surrender is attentiveness, or keeping your mind on God. Attentiveness, a practice of loving devotion, puts your life in perspective and lets you know that you are truly never alone. One form of attentiveness is *japa*, or continuously repeating the name of the divine as a mantra. A powerful example of this is Gandhi, who recited "*Ram*," a Sanskrit word for God. His mantra so filled his mind that, when he was shot by an assailant, he fell to the ground saying, "*Ram*."

DEVOTIONAL SALUTATION

We conclude this section with the practice of **namaste**. Namaste, a Sanskrit word, is a combination of two words: **namah** and **te**. Namah means "bow" and **te** means "to you." **Namaste** is translated as "I bow to you." Both greeting and meditation, it can be practiced when you are alone or with others. To perform it, bring your hands together in prayer, palms together and fingers pointing toward the sky. Place them in front of your heart, say "**Namaste**," close your eyes, and bow. Placing your hands over your heart chakra is an act of recognizing divine love. This position symbolizes a greeting between hearts. Alternatively, place your hands on top of your head, over your crown chakra, in an acknowledgment of the spiritual essence of the one you are bowing to. This transforms the greeting into one of devotion to the divine and is often interpreted as meaning "The divine in me acknowledges the divine in you."

Summary

Trauma and difficult transition are often interrelated. The aftermath of trauma can significantly alter how you live, and difficult life transitions can bring old trauma to the surface. Both are times when your relationship with the sacred becomes heightened, either as a resource for coping, a source of disconnect, or as a central aspect of your life.

Although early-life trauma may distort your experience of the sacred, coming to terms with sexual abuse and violence is often connected with a spiritual search and centering your life on the sacred. Likewise, healing from adult traumas is associated with involvement in religious and spiritual life or meditation practices that focus on accessing quiet inner states.

The yoga sutras help you to center life on the sacred and encourage dedication and persistence in meditation and prayer life. The sutras encourage you to ask for help from wise beings, living and deceased. They teach you to cultivate life-affirming attitudes to stabilize your mind. And perhaps most fundamental, the sutras counsel you to surrender your life, including troubles and successes, to the divine.

conclusion

My life is my message.

—Mahatma Gandhi

any great souls, known and unknown, who have experienced tremendous suffering have gone on to live exemplary lives. Mahatma Gandhi was one such individual. (In fact, the Sanskrit word *mahatma* means "great soul.") Like you, Mahatma Gandhi—who experienced racism, was beaten as a young attorney, and was imprisoned on four occasions—knew trauma. He did not let oppression define him, although undoubtedly those experiences informed his life's work. He relied on a yogic lifestyle, one that included periods of silence, study of sacred scriptures, and mantra recitation, for strength and sustenance. His unwavering spiritual practice supported his capacity to practice nonviolence, even at threat to his own life. He modeled that there is something more important to do with life than recoiling from it because of things that have happened. A beloved spiritual and political leader, Mahatma Gandhi was a champion of human equality and political independence for India. He taught us all that freedom is possible through nonviolent actions.

Your dedication to healing is a strong statement that acknowledges that even though traumas have touched you, you are taking back your life or perhaps finding your life for the first time. In doing so, you are standing up for the sacred nature of life. Yoga states that even if you were treated with disrespect, you attempt to be respectful to yourself and others. You embrace compassion, focus on life-affirming ideas, and declare "*neti, neti*" or "not this, not this" to thoughts that defile you or another person.

We are not minimizing the impact that trauma can have on your body and mind. However, you have chosen healing. Day by day you can vow to rise above the dark waters of ignorance and maltreatment. You can become like the beautiful lotus plant that symbolizes rebirth and divinity. The lotus grows in marshes and ponds. Its roots are in the mud, its stalk rises through the water, and it blooms above the water. This delicate flower offers the analogy that out of murky circumstances true spiritual beauty can be expressed. As Mahatma Gandhi did, you can set your sights on things that matter most to you.

At times you may not see your way. After all, old habits are hard to break. However, as Mahatma Gandhi said, freedom includes the freedom to make mistakes. Surely you've made some and will make some more. But you can learn and you can rise again. You lift yourself up whenever you go to your yoga mat, sit on your meditation cushion, breathe deeply, bow to the sacred, and give yourself over to your practice.

Your life is your message. Let it be one of hope, for your benefit and for the benefit of others. Like a lotus, which has exceptionally hearty seedpods that often plant themselves far from the source, you can spread the message that, in spite of it all, life is a blessing and can be lived that way.

bibliography

Abram, K. M., L. A. Teplin, D. R. Charles et al. 2004. "Post-Traumatic Stress Disorder and Trauma in Youth in Juvenile Detention." *Archives of General Psychiatry* 61, 403–410.

Ajaya, Swami. 1983. *Psychotherapy East and West: A Unifying Paradigm.* Honesdale, PA: The Himalayan International Institute.

Anodea, J. 1996. *Eastern Body, Western Mind.* Berkeley: Celestial Arts.

Badosi, A., L. Toribioz, and E. Garcia-Graui. 2008. "Traumatic Events and Tonic Immobility." *The Spanish Journal of Psychology* 11(2): 516–521.

Banks, S. M. and R. D. Kerns. 1996. "Explaining the High Rates of Depression in Chronic Pain: A Diathesis-Stress Framework." *Psychological Bulletin* 119: 95–110.

Begley, S. 2007. *Train Your Mind to Change Your Brain.* New York: Ballantine Books.

Besdine, R. 2011. "The Stigma Around Aging and Chronic Pain." *Huffington Post*, July 17, http.huffingtonpost.com/richard-w-besdine-md/aging-chronic-pain_b_905719.html.

Bierman, A. 2005. "The Effects of Childhood Maltreatment on Adult Religiosity and Spirituality: Rejecting God the Father Because of Abusive Fathers?" *The Journal for the Scientific Study of Religion* 44(3): 349–359.

Blanchard, E., E. J. Hickling, T. Galovski et al. 2002. "Emergency Room Vital Signs and PTSD in a Treatment Seeking Sample of Motor Vehicle Accident Survivors." *Journal of Traumatic Stress* 15(3): 199–204.

Burt, V. K. 2004 "Plotting the Course to Remission: The Search for Better Outcomes in the Treatment of Depression." *Journal of Clinical Psychiatry* 65(12): 20–5.

Carrión, V., B. Haas, A. Garrett et al. 2010. "Reduced Hippocampal Activity in Youth with Posttraumatic Stress Symptoms: An FMRI Study." *Journal of Pediatric Psychology* 35(5): 559–569.

Childre, D. and H. Martin. 1999. *The HeartMath Solution: The Institute of HeartMath's Revolutionary Program for Engaging the Power of the Heart's Intelligence*. New York: Harper Collins Publishers.

Cloitre, M., L. Cohen, and K. Koenen. 2006. *Treating Survivors of Childhood Abuse: Psychotherapy for the Interrupted Life*. New York: Guilford Publications, Inc.

Copeland, W., G. Keeler, A. Angold et al. 2007. "Traumatic Events and Posttraumatic Stress in Childhood." *Archives of General Psychiatry* 64(5): 577–584.

Cozolino, L. 2010. *The Neuroscience of Psychotherapy: Healing the Social Brain*. New York: W.W. Norton & Company.

Dale, S. and J. Daniel. 2011. "Spirituality/Religion as a Healing Pathway for Survivors of Sexual Violence" in *Surviving Sexual Violence: A Guide to Recovery*, edited by Thema Bryant-Davis. Lanham, MA: Rowman & Littlefield Publishers.

Desikachar, T. K. V. 1995. *The Heart of Yoga: Developing a Personal Practice*. Rochester, VA: Inner Traditions International.

Durgananda, Swami. 2002. *The Heart of Meditation: Pathways to a Deeper Experience.* South Falls, NY: SYDA Foundation.

Easwaran, E. 1994. *Take Your Time: Finding Balance in a Hurried World.* New York: Hyperion.

Elkins, D. N. 1995. "Psychotherapy and Spirituality: Toward a Theory of the Soul." *Journal of Humanistic Psychology* 35: 78–98.

Felitti V. J., R. F. Anda, D. Nordernberg et al. 1998. "Relationship of Childhood Abuse to Many of the Leading Causes of Death in Adults: The Adverse Childhood Experience (ACE) Study." *American Journal of Preventative Medicine* 14: 245–258.

Ferreira, V. M. and A. M. Sherman. 2007. "The Relationship of Optimism, Pain and Social Support to Well-Being in Older Adults with Osteoarthritis." *Aging Mental Health* 11(1): 89–98.

Finger, A. 2005. *Chakra Yoga: Balancing Energy for Physical, Spiritual, and Mental Well-Being.* Boston: Shambhala.

Finkelhor, D., H. Turner, and R. Ormrod, et al. 2009. "Children's Exposure to Violence: A Comprehensive National Survey." Office of Justice Programs and Delinquency Prevention: Washington, DC, www.ncjrs.gov/pdffiles1/ojjdp/227744.pdf.

Finkelhor, D., H. A. Turner, and S. L. Hamby. 2005. "The Victimization of Children and Youth: A Comprehensive, National Survey." *Child Maltreatment* 10(1): 5–25.

Gallop, G. and J. Maser. 1977. "Tonic Immobility: Evolutionary Underpinnings of Human Catalepsy and Catatonia." In *Psychopathology: Experimental Models,* edited by M. E. P. Seligman and J. D. Maser. San Francisco: W.H. Freeman.

Germer, C. 2009. *The Mindful Path to Self-Compassion.* New York: The Guilford Press.

Gilbert, P. 2010. *Compassion Focused Therapy: Distinctive Features.* New York: Routledge.

Glaister, J. A. and E. Abel. 2001. "Experiences of Women Healing from Childhood Sexual Abuse." *Archives of Psychiatric Nursing* 15(4): 188–194.

Greenberg, J., J. Porteus, L. Simon et al. 1995. "Evidence of a Terror-Management Function of Cultural Icons: The Effects of Mortality Salience on the Inappropriate Use of Cherished Cultural Symbols." *Personality and Social Psychology Bulletin* 21: 1221–1228.

Hanna, T. 1988 *Somatics: Reawakening the Mind's Control of Movement, Flexibility, and Health.* Cambridge: Da Capo Press.

Hari Dass, Baba. 1999. *The Yoga Sutras of Patanjali: A Study Guide for Book 1.* Santa Cruz: Sri Rama Publishing.

Herman, J. 1997. *Trauma and Recovery.* New York City: Basic Books.

Herman, J. 2007. "Shattered Shame States and Their Repair." Presented at The John Bowlby Memorial Conference. London, England. March 10.

Hickling, E. and E. Blanchard. 2006. *Overcoming the Trauma of Your Motor Vehicle Accident: A Cognitive-Behavioral Treatment Program Workbook.* New York: Oxford University Press.

Iwaniec, D., E. Larkin, and D. McSherry. July 2007. "Emotionally Harmful Parenting." *Child Care in Practice* 13(3): 203–220.

Iyengar, B. S. K. 1979. *Light on Yoga.* New York: Schocken Books.

Kane, D., S. E. Cheston, and R. Greer. 1993. "Perceptions of God by Survivors of Childhood Sexual Abuse: An Exploratory Study in an Under Researched Area." *Journal of Psychology and Theology* 21: 228–237.

Keating, Fr. T. 2010. *Centering Prayer: A Training Course for Opening to the Presence of God.* Boulder: Sounds True.

Kessler R. C., A. Sonnega, E. Bromet et al. 1995. "Post-traumatic Stress Disorder in the National Comorbidity Survey." *Archives of General Psychiatry* 52(12): 1048–60.

Killingsworth, M. and D. Gilbert. 2010. "A Wandering Mind Is an Unhappy Mind." *Science* 330(6006): 932.

Knapik, G., D. S. Martsolf, C. Draucker et al. 2010. "Attributes of Spirituality Described by Survivors of Sexual Violence." *The Qualitative Report* 15(3): 644–657.

Kolodiejchuk, B. ed. 2007. *Mother Teresa: Come Be My Light*. New York: Random House.

Konstan, D. 2001. *Pity Transformed*. London: Duckworth.

Lakkireddy, D., J. Pillarisetti, D. Atkins et al. 2011. "Impact of Yoga on Arrhythmia Burden and Quality of Life in Patients with Symptomatic Paroxysmal Atrial Fibrillation: The Yoga My Heart Study." *Journal of the American College of Cardiology* 57(14s1): E129.

LaMothe, R. 1998. "Sacred Objects as Vital Objects: Transitional Objects Reconsidered." *Journal of Psychology and Theology* 26: 159–167.

Lanius, R., E. Vermetten, and C. Pain. 2010. *The Impact of Early Life Trauma on Health and Disease: The Hidden Epidemic*. Cambridge: Cambridge University Press.

Lepine, J. P. and M. Briley. 2004 "The Epidemiology of Pain and Depression." *Human Psychopharmacology: Clinical & Experimental* 19(S1): S3–7.

Levine, P. 2010. *In an Unspoken Voice*. Berkeley: North Atlantic Books.

Lutz, A., J. Brefczynski-Lewis, T. Johnstone et al. 2008. "Regulation of the Neural Circuitry of Emotion by Compassion Meditation: Effects of Meditative Expertise." *PLOS ONE* 3(3): e1897, doi:10.1371/journal.pone.0001897.

Maclean, K., E. Ferrer, S. Aichele et al. 2010. "Intensive Meditation Training Improves Perceptual Discrimination and Sustained Attention." *Psychological Science* 21(6): 829–839.

Martinez, J., A. Garakani, H. Kaufman et al. 2010. "Heart Rate and Blood Pressure Changes During Autonomic Nervous System Challenge in Panic Disorder Patients." *Psychosomatic Medicine Journal* 72(5): 442–449.

Merton, T. 1969. *Contemplative Prayer*. New York: Herder & Herder.

Miller, L. R. and A. Cano. 2009. "CoMorbid Chronic Pain and Depression: Who Is at Risk?" *Psychology Faculty Research Publications* Paper 14, http://digitalcommons.wayne.edu/psychfrp/ 14.

201

Morin, R. 2011. "The Difficult Transition from Military to Civilian Life." Washington, D.C., Pew Research Center. December 12, http.pewsocial trends.org/2011/12/08/the-difficult-transition-from-military-to-civilian-life.

The National Intimate Partner and Sexual Violence Survey. Centers for Disease Control and Prevention. December 14, 2011.

Neimark, J. 2007. "The Optimism Revolution." *Psychology Today* May/June: 88–94.

Newberg, A. and M. Waldman. 2009. *How God Changes Your Brain.* New York: Ballantine Books.

Nhat Hanh, T. 2009. *You Are Here: Discovering the Magic of the Present Moment.* Boston: Shambhala.

Nisargadatta, M., translated by M. Frydman. 1990. *I Am That.* San Diego: Acorn Press.

Osborne, A., editor. 1972. *The Collected Works of Ramana Maharshi.* New Beach, ME: Samuel Weiser, Inc.

Pargament, K. I. 1997. *The Psychology of Religion and Coping: Theory, Research, Practice.* New York: Guilford Press.

Park, C. L. 2005. "Religion and Meaning." In *Handbook of the Psychology of Religion and Spirituality,* edited by R. F. Paloutzian and C. L. Park. New York: Guilford Press.

Porges, S. 2011. *The Polyvagal Theory.* New York: W.W. Norton & Company.

Rama, Swami, R. Ballentine, and Swami Ajaya. 1976. *Yoga and Psychotherapy: The Evolution of Consciousness.* Honesdale: The Himalayan International Institute of Yoga Science and Philosophy.

Rosenthal, J., S. Grosswald, R. Ross et al. 2011. "Effects of Transcendental Meditation in Veterans of Operation Enduring Freedom and Operation Iraqi Freedom with Post-Traumatic Stress Disorder: A Pilot study." *Military Medicine* 176: 626–630.

Ryan, P. L. 1998. "An Exploration of the Spirituality of Fifty Women Who Survived Childhood Violence." *Journal of Transpersonal Psychology* 30: 87–102.

Scaer, R. 2005. *The Trauma Spectrum: Hidden Wounds and Human Resilience.* New York: W.W. Norton.

Schuster, M. A., B. C. Stein, L. H. Joycox et al. 2001. "A National Survey of Stress Reactions After the September 11, 2001 Terrorist Attacks." *New England Journal of Medicine* 345: 1507–1512.

Shaw, A., S. Joseph, and P. A. Linley. 2005. "Religion, Spirituality, and Posttraumatic Growth: A Systematic Review." *Mental Health, Religion & Culture* 8(1): 1–11.

Smith, M. and L. Kelly. 2001. "The Journey of Recovery After a Rape Experience." *Issues in Mental Health Nursing* 22(4): 337–352.

Stiles, M. 2002. *Yoga Sutras of Patanjali.* Boston: Red Wheel/Weiser, LLC.

Stone, D. 2009. "One Nation Under God." *Newsweek Survey* April 6.

Streeter, C., T. H. Whitfield, L. Owen et al. 2010. "Effects of Yoga Versus Walking on Mood, Anxiety and Brain GABA Levels: A Randomized Controlled MRS Study." *The Journal of Alternative and Complementary Medicine* 16(11): 1145–52.

Tigunait, P. R. 2011. "The Legacy of the Sages." *Yoga International Journal* 116: 34–41.

Trapper, B. 2009. *Identifying and Recovering from Psychological Trauma.* New York: Gordian Knot Books.

van der Kolk, B. 2010. *Neuroscience and Trauma Theory.* Seminar on DVD. One hour and twenty-four minutes. Item # ZNV042980. Premier Education Solutions: Boston. DVD.

van der Kolk, B. 2011. *Bessel van der Kolk's 22nd Annual Trauma Conference—Psychological Trauma: Neuroscience, Attachment and Therapeutic Interventions.* Seminar on DVD. Four hours and forty-six minutes. Item # ZNV043895. Premier Education Solutions: Boston. DVD.

Wachholtz, A. B. and K. I. Pargament. 2005. "Is Spirituality a Critical Ingredient of Meditation? Comparing the Effects of Spiritual Meditation, Secular Meditation, and Relaxation on Spiritual, Psychological, Cardiac, and Pain Outcomes." *Journal of Behavioral Medicine* 28(4): 369–384.

Wachholtz, A. B. and K. I. Pargament. 2008. "Migraines and Meditation: Does Spirituality Matter?" *Journal of Behavioral Medicine* 31(4): 351–366.

Wiens, S. 2006. "Subliminal Emotion Perception in Brain Imaging: Findings, Issues, and Recommendations." *Progress in Brain Research* 156: 105–121.

Yogananda, P. 1946. *The Autobiography of a Yogi*. New York: The Philosophical Library.

Zeidan, F., K. T. Martucci, R. A. Kraft et al. 2011. "Brain Mechanisms Supporting the Modulation of Pain by Mindfulness Meditation." *The Journal of Neuroscience* 31(14): 5540–5548.

Zucker, T., F. Muench, R. Gevirtz. 2009. "The Effects of Respiratory Sinus Arrhythmia Biofeedback on Heart Rate Variability and Posttraumatic Stress Disorder Symptoms: A Pilot Study." *Applied Psychophysiology and Biofeedback Journal* 34(2): 135–143.

Mary NurrieStearns, LCSW, RYT, is a psychotherapist and yoga teacher with a counseling practice in Tulsa, OK. She is author of numerous articles on psychospiritual growth, coeditor of the book Soulful Living, coauthor of the book Yoga for Anxiety, and has produced DVDs on yoga for anxiety and emotional trauma. She leads transformational meditation and yoga retreats and teaches seminars across the United States.

Rick NurrieStearns, is a meditation teacher, coauthor of the book Yoga for Anxiety, and coeditor of Soulful Living. For ten years he was the publisher of Personal Transformation, a magazine focusing on psychospiritual growth. He has been immersed in consciousness studies and yoga practices for nearly four decades. In 2009 he survived a nearfatal airplane crash that resulted in chronic pain. He credits the practice of meditation with helping him navigate through extreme pain and the journey of recovery.

Visit the NurrieStearns online at www.personaltransformation.com.